Patient and Staff Voi
Primary Care

. . . a fascinating read and a rich source, which will be of value to a wide audience—to medical historians interested in general practice and the history of the National Health Service; to social scientists studying illness behaviour and 'pathways to the doctor'; to anyone interested in the social history of Glasgow.

—Malcolm Nicolson PhD Hon FRCPSG
Emeritus Professor of the History of Medicine
University of Glasgow

This unique work represents the recording and analysis of oral history interviews conducted by the pioneering general practitioner Dr Hetty Ockrim with over seventy patients, as well as office staff and members of the nursing team, between 1989 and 1992 in her former practice in the Ibrox/Govan areas of Glasgow, places of significant socio-economic deprivation. Her focus in undertaking this study was on personal and social, rather than just clinical, issues. The interviews are accompanied by background and commentary for the study, reflecting the full breadth of general practice. Many of the interviewees had memories stretching back before the NHS, providing a unique historical perspective of service development, as well as invaluable directions for improving current and future general practice.

Key Features

- Provides a historical context for the developments in health over several decades prior to the study
- Shows how oral history methods have increasingly been used in medical history research and explores the benefits of this approach
- Covers many of the themes of the oral history which enabled and encouraged patients to comment on what was important to them in their encounters with health care
- Follows the increasing acceptance of women in medicine, demonstrating how women doctors were viewed by patients within the practice compared to changes in wider society
- Presents a 'history from below', using voices that are not normally heard in the medical discourse, illustrating the importance of the doctor–patient interface

Supporting a wider understanding of what patient narratives can tell us about the delivery of health care from the perspective of the patients, the front-line users of health services, the book shows how oral history can provide an understanding of health care more broadly, key at a time when social inequality is once again widening in many regions.

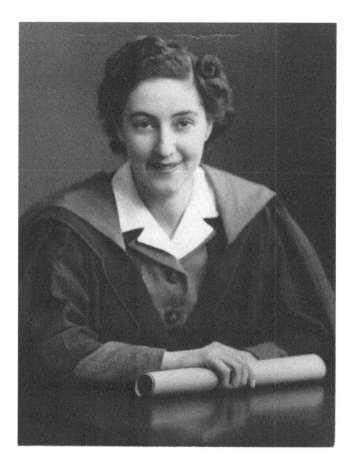

Dr Hetty Ockrim, MB ChB, Graduation, January 1943

Patient and Staff Voices in Primary Care
Learning from Dr Ockrim and Her Glasgow Medical Practice

Kenneth E Collins MB ChB MPhil PhD FRCGP

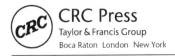

CRC Press
Taylor & Francis Group
Boca Raton London New York

CRC Press is an imprint of the
Taylor & Francis Group, an **informa** business

First edition published 2023
by CRC Press
6000 Broken Sound Parkway NW, Suite 300, Boca Raton, FL 33487–2742

and by CRC Press
4 Park Square, Milton Park, Abingdon, Oxon, OX14 4RN

CRC Press is an imprint of Taylor & Francis Group, LLC

© 2023 Kenneth E. Collins

ISBN: 9781032439013 (hbk)
ISBN: 9781032432137 (pbk)
ISBN: 9781003369301 (ebk)

DOI: 10.1201/9781003369301

Typeset in Minion
by Apex CoVantage, LLC

Contents

Foreword

Patient and Staff Voices in Primary Care: Learning from Dr Ockrim and Her Glasgow Medical Practice is a remarkable, indeed possibly a unique, piece of historiography. Between 1989 and 1992, Dr Hetty Ockrim, newly retired as a general practitioner, conducted oral history interviews with many of her former patients, as well as some members of the administrative and nursing staff. Her focus was on personal and social, rather than just clinical, issues. The transcripts of these interviews have been skilfully edited, arranged thematically with detailed commentary, by her son, Dr Kenneth E Collins, following his retirement from the same Ibrox/ Govan practice.

Originally, the history of medicine was written only by doctors, who wrote mainly about the doings of other doctors and, sometimes, of medical scientists. The patient was substantially absent from this literature, appearing only as the unspeaking object of diagnosis or therapy. It was not until the 1970s that a historiography developed that was about medicine but did not wholly derive from the medical profession. Health and health care were recognised as aspects of humanity's story that were too important to be left entirely to doctors. Matters such as public health, pandemics, women's health, child-rearing, and so forth, began to be addressed by social and economic historians. And historians began to realise the importance of giving a voice to the patient.

As Roy Porter argued, in his seminal article 'The Patient's View: Doing Medical History from Below' (*Theory and Society*, 1985), an account of medicine that is centred solely on the physician runs the risk of serious historical distortion 'for it takes two to make a medical encounter'. Clinical medicine is, to a large degree, a secondary phenomenon, substantially dependent on decisions made by lay people. It is they who first identify the presence of illness and only subsequently may seek professional advice. Answers to the central question, 'Should I see a doctor?' are structured not only by individual decision-making processes but also by the beliefs and attitudes about health and medicine, which are prevalent in the community that each sufferer inhabits.

Oral historiography has proven to be a very effective method of investigating attitudes to health and health care among those who would not otherwise be heard, of giving the patient a voice. It is, however, a methodology which requires tact and sensitivity if it is to be done well. It is a credit to Dr Ockrim, and indeed to Dr Collins, that they both took the course in oral historiography of medicine organised by Professor Paul Thompson, University of Essex, recognised as a leading pioneer of the technique in Britain. Dr Ockrim shows herself to be an empathetic, non-judgemental and, to an extent, self-effacing interviewer, with an unrivalled knowledge of the Govan area, its issues of socio-economic deprivation, as well as its strong sense of community. A great strength of the interview material is that it is obvious that she has the confidence of her interviewees, having been, in many cases, their family doctor, often for more than one generation. She understands how social and personal factors interact with issues of health and welfare. There is an enjoyable irony in the fact that such an effective demonstration of the value of a departure from the physician-centred approach should be accomplished by a physician.

We are greatly in Dr Collins's debt. He has provided us with a fascinating read and a rich source, which will be of value to a wide audience—to medical historians interested in general practice and the history of the National Health Service, to social scientists studying illness behaviour and pathways to the doctor or urban health issues more broadly, to anyone interested in the social history of Glasgow. It is also a valuable contribution to the history of female entry into the medical profession and of the Jewish community in Glasgow.

Malcolm Nicolson PhD Hon FRCPSG
Emeritus Professor of the History of Medicine
University of Glasgow

Acknowledgements

My grateful thanks to all the patients and staff members of the Midlock Medical Centre who agreed to be interviewed by Dr Ockrim between 1989 and 1992, and permitted me to use material from their interviews in building the story of general practice in the Ibrox and Govan areas of Glasgow. Thanks are due to the Wellcome Foundation, who provided the funding for the interview process and for the transcribing of all the interviews. Thanks also to Sandra Grant, who transcribed the testimonies over many hundreds of hours, catching so beautifully the idiom of the spoken words.

Thanks to Professor Arthur McIvor of the Scottish Oral History Archives at the University of Strathclyde for agreeing to store the original interview tapes and for arranging their digitisation. Under the terms of the original agreement with the interviewees, access to the tapes is strictly limited and the copyright is held on behalf of the interviewees by me and the current doctors at the Midlock Medical Centre whose co-operation in the thirty years since the study began is much appreciated.

My especial thanks to Professor Malcolm Nicolson, Dr Hannah-Louise Clark and Professor Jude Robinson for their wise counsel and guidance during the writing of this work. I have found the Centre for the History of Medicine a safe haven for medical history research and writing for many years.

Short extracts of this study have been presented at conferences in London (British Medical Association); Edinburgh (British Society for the History of Medicine); Halkidiki, Greece (Physician Health); Jerusalem (UNESCO Bioethics); and Auckland (Australia and New Zealand Society for the History of Medicine). These presentations followed themes of women in medicine, the beginnings of the National Health Service and resilience as an essential character trait in medical practice. An essay which outlined some of the content of the interviews was awarded the Rose Prize by the Royal College of General Practitioners and the Master of the Worshipful Society of Apothecaries in May 2019. Two related papers were published in the *Journal of Medical Biography* and the *British Medical Journal*.

Author

Kenneth E Collins MB ChB FRCGP MPhil (Medical Law and Ethics) PhD (Medical History) is Senior Research Fellow, Centre for the History of Medicine, University of Glasgow, and currently Visiting Professor, History of Medicine, Hebrew University of Jerusalem, Israel.

Abbreviations

ARP	Air Raid Precautions
BMA	British Medical Association
BMJ	*British Medical Journal*
DSS	Department of Social Security
GPFC	General Practice Finance Corporation
HCP	Health Care Practitioner
MVLS	Medical, Veterinary and Life Sciences
NHI	National Health Insurance
NHS	National Health Service
RCGP	Royal College of General Practitioners
SAMH	Scottish Association of Mental Health
SOHC	Scottish Oral History Centre
TB	Tuberculosis
UNESCO	United Nations Scientific Educational and Cultural Organisation

1

Introduction

This work represents the recording and analysis of oral history interviews conducted between 1989 and 1992 in one practice in the Ibrox/Govan areas of Glasgow, places of significant socio-economic deprivation. My mother, Dr Ockrim, who had just retired as Senior Partner in the practice, conducted the interviews of over seventy patients as well as key members of the practice's office staff and nursing teams, besides providing background and commentary for the study based on her extensive experience of general practice. Many of the interviewees had memories stretching back before the NHS and could describe the practice of Dr Stevan George, who had founded the practice in 1924, and how care was delivered at the time. I was also a principal in her practice from 1977 till 2009 and knew most of the interviewees as patients also.

This work will show how oral history can provide an understanding of health care and its delivery in an inner-city practice, significantly affected by social and economic deprivation. Patient views describe historic health care issues which tells of the past as well as indicating future needs.

Frequently mentioned factors include the major impact of the creation of the National Health Service, how patients' respect for the doctor's authority impacts their health care, how stigma and marginalisation affected the health and welfare of patients and issues related to women and medicine. Some of these themes are universal and speak for communities and societies far beyond Glasgow, where people describe past struggles for access to medical care, free at the point of contact, understanding from their family doctor and full coverage from specialised medical services and hospital inpatient treatment.

The book uses oral history testimonies to present a history from below using voices that are not normally heard in the medical discourse. The use of oral history will enable the understanding of the following themes:

1. Provide a historical context for the developments in health over several decades prior to the study. To do this will require an understanding of how the practice was formed and operated prior to the National Health Service and how delivery of care within the practice was seen by the patients to change after 1948.
2. Follow the increasing acceptance of women in medicine, showing how women doctors were viewed by patients within the practice, along with changes in the wider society.

DOI: 10.1201/9781003369301-1

3. Understand what oral history can tell us about the delivery of health care from the perspective of the patients, the users of the health services, illustrating the doctor–patient interface.

I will show how oral history methods have increasingly been used in medical history research and will explore the benefits of this approach. I will also show how this study adds to the growing body of material on the history of general medical practice in Britain through patient narratives, as mediated by one of their own family doctors.[1] This account of the health care of patients in one urban practice allows for their own understandings in the telling of the story. I will show that the choice of the retired doctor interviewing former patients gives a different perspective on oral medical history compared with previous studies where interviews of general practitioners or patients were conducted by social scientists.[2] When I discovered the interviewer's 'Letters to No-One' after her death, it became possible for the oral histories to form part of a narrative illuminating not just the practice of medicine in one area of Glasgow but also the remarkable practitioner who conducted the interviews.

The study generated a considerable amount of quantitative data. In 2000, the *British Medical Journal* printed an article showing that qualitative research, such as in verbatim notes or transcribed recordings of interviews, can produce 'vast amounts of data'.[3] I have followed this approach which indicates that the analytical process begins during data collection, allowing the researcher to go back and refine questions, develop hypotheses and pursue emerging avenues of inquiry in further depth. It also allows the use of paper systems, which may be considered old-fashioned and laborious but can help the researcher to develop an intimate knowledge of the data. This approach can yield issues which may be unlikely to arise in the clinical encounter.[4]

In 2014, with concern about the long-term survival of the audiotapes, the oral history recordings and the transcripts were deposited at the Scottish Oral History Centre (SOHC) which was established at the University of Strathclyde, Glasgow, in 1995, and is involved in a wide range of teaching, research and outreach activities designed primarily to encourage the use of 'best practice' oral history methodology in Scotland.[5]

Thus, this study derives from three separate elements. The first is the major collection of oral history interviews recorded by Dr Ockrim between 1989 and 1992 following her retiral from general practice in the Midlock Medical Centre and its detailed analysis in the production of this book. She was keen to remain intellectually active and still maintain an interest in medicine, and she was enthusiastic when I suggested the idea of an oral history project to her. The interviewer was aware of the risks of being the dominant individual in the telling of the patients' stories. Great care was taken to ensure that she was mainly the silent facilitator for the accounts which emerged. For many patients, memories extended back to the years before the formation of the National Health Service in 1948 and, for a few, back as far or even further than the 1930s.

The second element follows Dr Ockrim's assiduous collection of notes, and some of this commentary forms an important part of the study. We have her records of impressions of practice over her decades in medicine, first as an obstetrician/gynaecologist in hospital and then as a general practitioner, firstly in Cessnock Street (1946–1987) and finally in Midlock Street (1987–1989). There are further notes in a card index of the interviews and on the questionnaires, which accompanied each patient interview. This formed a useful guide to the importance of the testimony.

Because it contains much confidential material, it has only been used in exceptional, and clearly noted and attributed, circumstances. These notes were finally supplemented by the 'Letters to No-one' which described the retirement process as she saw it. Handwritten over six months during 1987, these three letters illustrate her feelings at this important milestone in her life and add a fascinating additional dimension to the oral history study itself. The letters were only discovered after her death in August 2007. They are a unique window into her mind.

In the final element, we cover many of the themes of the oral history which lets her patients comment on what was important to them in their encounter with health care in the Ibrox and Govan areas of Glasgow. This is a rich seam of oral history which deserves a wide audience—especially for health care professionals and the consumers of their services. Next, we will try to understand the individual, and her personality, behind the interviews and the author of the 'Letters to No-one'. She faced prejudices as a woman on her way into medicine. There was family opposition to her entry into medical school in 1938. As a female medical graduate in 1943, she had to face prejudice, often from patients as much as from senior colleagues.

ETHICAL APPROVAL

I first applied for ethical approval for writing up the oral history project in 2007, as regulations had been much more informal at the time the interviews were conducted. On the 8th of August 2007, the Research Ethics R&D Directorate of NHS Greater Glasgow and Clyde gave a favourable opinion on 'An Oral History of one urban General medical practice based on interviews with patients producing a narrative of the delivery of care measured against developments in the life story of the individual, their family and carers'.[6]

Their only stipulation was that if any further interviews were contemplated, the consent form should be amended to include specific consent to tape the interviews and for publication of the data. It was indicated that the favourable opinion was for the duration of the research.

When the current work began, it was agreed to revisit the ethical issues. The opinion of Professor Arthur McIvor of the Scottish Oral History Centre at the University of Strathclyde, where the interviews, now digitised, are held, ruled favourably on ethical approval, counselling only that care should be taken to preserve anonymity and to avoid quoting material which could prejudice individuals living or dead. Consequently, I have used a simple letter code for the quotes except for two interviewees who have waived anonymity. Professor McIvor's opinion was also accepted by the College of Ethics of Glasgow University MVLS Faculty.[7]

THE FAMILY DOCTOR

When Ronald Gibson published his book on general practice in 1981, he described the role of the family doctor in the following terms.[8]

Traditionally in Britain the doctor first consulted in an illness is known as a general practitioner. . . . The doctor responds to patients' calls either by treatment in the surgery or by visiting at home. He may be the only doctor involved in the illness or he may have to arrange admission to hospital, taking over care again when the patient is back home. It is likely that a GP will be a doctor to all the members of the family and will look after them throughout his practising years, being involved in many important events in their lives, including births, marriages and deaths. He becomes used to giving advice with very little relation to health in the strict sense and is regarded as a counsellor and friend as well as a doctor.

This narrative has been modified with the passage of time, as more modern working practices have emerged and with the increasing presence of female doctors. However, the doctor remains at the centre of the key moments of life and usually directs the care needed at all stages of illness.

This book has broken new ground in recording the history of general practice in its comprehensive approach to patient care through the interaction of doctor and patient. In considering primary care as a specialist entity, many of the different aspects of what constitutes best practice have also been a fruitful field of study. In his book *Talking with Patients*, Philip Myerscough emphasised the importance of language, both spoken and silent, and body language in encouraging the patient to disclose all the information the doctor requires. This includes conveying a sense of available time and ensuring that the patient has said everything they needed to express.[9]

A qualitative study was conducted on the views of patients living in Drumchapel in 1991, an area of high socio-economic deprivation in Glasgow.[10] Key issues centred round the GPs' competence and ability to explain things clearly and in an understandable way. Also important was empathy or 'caring' which related to patients feeling valued, feeling listened to by the doctor and being able to talk and that the doctor understood 'the bigger picture'.[11]

Valerie Yow notes that in the early days of oral history, there was no acknowledgement about the effect on the interviewer of carrying out the interviews.[12] Yow considers the interviewer's motives as important and notes the intrusion of the interviewer's views into the process. We have noted only two instances of this in the hundreds of hours of testimony. In defence of the National Health Service, Dr Ockrim took issue with a participant's views of the benefits of American medicine, and she challenged an interviewee on their objection to immigrant Pakistanis speaking in their native language in the waiting room.

In its first years, oral history was often criticised for presenting the selective memories of those interviewed. It is acknowledged that the passage of time and the way in which the story is heard, how it is to be recorded and who will eventually access it, are all factors which may affect the story. In addition, there is said to be a tendency for patients to look at the past through the prism of their present experiences. However, studies, such as this account of the history of one general practitioner and her medical practice in Glasgow, have much to contribute to our understanding of the delivery of medical care before and after the establishment of the National Health Service.

DR OCKRIM: A BRIEF BIOGRAPHY

Hetty Brenda Ockrim was born in Merryland Street, in Govan, on the 23rd of August 1919, at the home of her Ockrim grandparents. The building, a stone villa, faced the St Francis Nursing Home which was to be such an important part of her medical life. Her four grandparents had arrived in Glasgow in the 1890s, part of the large wave of Jewish emigration from the Russian Empire, stimulated by the poverty and anti-Semitism in the Pale of Settlement which saw millions of Jews settle in the United States, Britain and Western Europe.

The first 10 years of her life were spent in Abbotsford Place in the Glasgow Gorbals. Though the Gorbals was already becoming a slum area by the 1920s, Abbotsford Place retained a certain gentility where the more prosperous of the neighbourhood's population lived. She attended Abbotsford Primary School before going on to Hutchesons' Grammar School for Girls.

As a teenager, Dr Ockrim had already decided that she wanted a career in medicine. Her younger sisters were to become accountants, while her younger brother, Jack, eventually gave up his medical studies just a year or so before the finals because of increasing mental health problems. The availability of places at the large Scottish university medical schools, the availability of Carnegie grants for needy students,[13] lower class fees than in the English medical schools and the option of the three Scottish extra-mural medical schools were all powerful attractions. While the extra-mural schools, Anderson's College and St Mungo's College in Glasgow and the Medical School of the Royal Colleges of Physicians and Surgeons in Edinburgh, led to the Triple Qualification rather than the MB ChB of the universities, this still led to the desired place on the medical register.[14]

The major movement of Jews into medicine in Scotland, especially with the rise of the first generation to be born in Scotland, was essentially a male phenomenon. Even by 1938, the number of Jewish women in medicine in Scotland was just a bare handful, and her father, Louis, felt that the medical profession was not one for a young Jewish girl. He, therefore, insisted that she choose a different course, which she dutifully did. She was accepted to study metallurgy at Glasgow University beginning in October 1938. Before starting university, speaking fluent French, she accompanied her father on a six-week trip to Paris, ostensibly for his business, but in reality, trying to arrange a permit for a stateless relative to enter Britain.

Most science courses, including medicine, had a basic science first year, including botany, biology, physics and chemistry, and this allowed flexibility of entrance to the more specialised subjects the following year. At the end of the first year, she made enquiries at the Medical Faculty, without telling her parents, and was accepted to enter the second year of the medical course. I don't know how the news was received, but it was obvious in later years just how proud her parents were of her care and compassion, and her remarkable energy which informed all that she did. Her parents were quickly reconciled to her devotion to medicine and were loyal patients of her practice all through their long lifetimes.

By the time Dr Ockrim entered the medical course, there was a significant group of female medical students, and she had many role models who had helped shape the role of women in medicine. Nevertheless, women were a minority in the medical profession, and most of the population might never have encountered one. Indeed, the proportion of women at the University of Glasgow had not changed in the years after World War I, remaining just over 10%.[15] Even as late as 1987, it was still being said that equality of access to medical schools had not led to equality of access to senior hospital appointments.[16]

The experience of being thwarted in her first year at university from embarking on the course of her choice and the action she took to put her career on track gave her a rare understanding of people trying to follow their dreams, and her ability to counsel people at the crossroads of life became legendary. Her studies were pursued enthusiastically, and she graduated in January 1943, followed by her first house jobs at the Glasgow Royal Infirmary. She often talked with much affection about her surgical residency under Professor John (Pop) Burton, holder of the St Mungo Chair at the University of Glasgow. Her plans were to go into obstetrics and gynaecology, but she was sympathetic to the plight of local doctors, unable to arrange locum cover for holiday breaks during the war, as so many doctors were with the British Army in different locations around the globe.

She spent some months working in Blantyre, then a small mining town not far from Glasgow. It was a rapid introduction to life in the community. There were mining accidents and the full range of medical conditions to treat in wartime conditions. She coped well with the work, and a reference from the practice doctor, Dr Arthur Gordon, related this:

> Dr Ockrim had the difficulty of being the first lady doctor in the practice and the way in which she not only overcame certain prejudices but won over these people, is in itself a testament to her abilities. The practice is a varied one with industrial and residential patients. Dr Ockrim made herself accepted by all and esteemed by them. In her work she was most diligent and applied herself not exclusively to the medical work proper but also to the ancillary tasks which beset general practice. She was a good clinician, sound in her diagnosis and treatment, and always anxious to learn and improve where possible.[17]

She worked next as a senior house officer and then registrar in Obstetrics and Gynaecology at the Elsie Inglis Hospital in Edinburgh, and the story of Elsie Maud Inglis was a continuing inspiration to her with her innovative medical work, her suffragist activity and her founding the Scottish Women's Hospitals during World War I. After this short spell in Edinburgh, she was ready for career development at the Glasgow Royal Infirmary and the Royal Samaritan Hospital for Women. In early 1946, as she neared the end of a first stage of obstetrics and gynaecology training, she received two references. Professor John Burton commented that she was 'a first-class diagnostician and a very safe anaesthetist'. In a more detailed reference from her current consultant, Dr Donald McIntyre, Glasgow University Lecturer in Gynaecology, wrote this on 15th October 1945:

> she was unsparing in the energy she devotes to her work, and she is held in the highest esteem by both parents and nursing staff. She has had the opportunity of special instruction in anaesthetics by the visiting anaesthetist and has proved herself a safe and competent anaesthetist.[18]

This was a skill she would employ in the early post-war years in conducting more complicated home deliveries.

However, her plans to continue her specialisation suddenly changed after meeting an ex-army doctor who was to become her husband. Dr David Collins had been born in London in February 1912 to a Jewish immigrant family from Ukraine. The family had moved to Glasgow just a few weeks later, in April 1912, where his father set up what became a significant textile business. David was the first, and only one, of his siblings to study at university, and he, too, had been set on a medical career. After graduation in 1939, his first medical work was at Blawarthill Hospital in Clydebank.

He was working at Blawarthill during the devastating Clydebank Blitz, when two massive air raids by the Luftwaffe took place on two successive nights in March 1941. The town suffered extensive destruction. Tens of thousands were made homeless, and there were 1,200 deaths with around a thousand seriously injured and many more with lighter levels of injury. There was extensive industrial damage to Clydebank's shipbuilding and other heavy industries, but the housing loss led to mass evacuation, the only British town that had to be evacuated due to enemy action. Blawarthill Hospital was first in line for casualties from the German air raids. A reference by its Medical Officer Dr W H Stirling Armstrong noted this on 18th August 1941:

> during his term as Resident Medical Officer the severe air raids of March occurred when 120 odd casualties were admitted. I am proud to testify to his devotion to duty and courage and to the creditable manner he performed his many duties during a period of great difficulty and tensions.[19]

After a year as a medical recruitment officer based at Rouken Glen Park just south of Glasgow, he joined the British 8th Army invasion of North Africa at the end of 1942 in the Operation Torch campaign. He was a field general practitioner based near the Algerian town of Bône (now Annaba) and was in an army unit which followed the invasion of Italy, spending time in both Rome and Florence, before returning to Glasgow after being demobbed at the end of 1945. When Drs David and Hetty met, they clearly made a great impression on each other. He could not believe at first that the young woman he was meeting was an obstetrician, but it was not long before they decided to enter general practice together. General practice had been a popular career choice for women for more than thirty years, and more women were becoming partners in practices.[20]

There were many young doctors returning home after the war, and army doctors who had seen active service over the previous six or seven years did not find it easy to buy a practice in 1946. Dr David had the advantage that, as he had joined up early and had worked with casualties during the Blitz, he was amongst the first to be demobbed. No doubt there were memories of the rush of demobbed doctors after World War I scrambling for practices, and he would have felt that there was no time to be lost.[21]

Dr Ockrim was then working at Glasgow's Royal Samaritan Hospital for Women where the consultant gynaecologist Dr Albert (Bert) Sharman was based. Bert Sharman (1903–1970) was one of the most distinguished gynaecologists of his generation.[22] An accomplished speaker and author of many textbooks, he was also an innovative inventor. Sharman had a medical friend in Ibrox, Dr Stevan George, who was expressing an interest in leaving Britain and his practice in Glasgow before the start of the National Health Service. They had been at university around the same time and would also have had regular professional contacts.

Sharman arranged for Dr George to meet with Drs Hetty Ockrim and David Collins, and by February 1946, they had bought the practice, and Dr Collins was working at 2 Cessnock Street. There was a short period of overlap as Dr George finished his work and introduced the new doctor to his patients, and Dr Collins was joined just a few months later by Dr Ockrim who arrived at the practice in June. They were married on 12th November 1946. There was family support to help them buy the practice, as was the custom in pre-NHS days. Friends' families also joined the practice at the time. One study participant claimed this:

> remember how it came about. It came about when David started, and his father started with my father and Louis Ockrim went and chatted to all his friends and said, 'Right, we're setting up a Practice'.
>
> (YT)

Drs David and Hetty took over the large ground-floor flat at the corner of Cessnock Street and Paisley Road West, situated directly across the road from the Cessnock Street subway station. They kept the resident caretaker who occupied some ground-floor rooms with additional accommodation in the basement.

After the National Health Service began the practice, population regularly numbered around 9,500. This size practice was normally served by four doctors, and consequently, a third partner, Dr Ian Russell, joined the practice in 1949, in addition to the regular appointment of a practice assistant. The practice continued with four doctors until the 1980s.[23] I joined the practice as an assistant in November 1976 and became a partner in the following April. Dr Barry Adams-Strump was at first a locum for Dr David following his stroke in 1978 and became a partner some months later when it was clear that Dr David would not be able to return to work. Dr Christine Grieve was appointed as an additional partner in 1986 just before the practice moved to the Midlock Medical Centre in Midlock Street, and Dr Ken O'Neill replaced Dr Russell in 1987. When Dr Ockrim retired in September 1989, she was replaced by Dr Alison Thomson.

The Letters to No-One

Dr Ockrim faced the prospect of retirement with some trepidation, and we discussed some options which would ease the transition from the active and bustling life of an inner-city general practitioner into more traditional retirement pursuits. It had become the norm for many general practitioners facing an increasingly intrusive NHS bureaucracy to retire around the age of 60 years. Dr Ockrim was not ready to leave her work at that stage, although she did stop her obstetrics work, then based in the General Practitioner Unit at the Southern General Hospital. She continued to practice till just after her 70th birthday, and it was only the discovery of a collection of letters in her desk after her death eighteen years later that gave an insight into her mood and feeling of that time.

There were three letters in an envelope with the words 'Letters to No-one' on the outside. These letters formed part of a presentation I made at the International Conference on Physician Health, sponsored by the Medical Associations of Britain, Canada and the United States of America in September 2014, in a session titled 'Planning Well for Senior Choices'. The conference was centred round physician wellbeing and the milestones and transitions in life which could affect it. One of these milestones was retirement, and many papers addressed the characteristics of personal resilience, physical strength and health.

An important part of this conference was the reflective session at the end of each day. The chairman of this session, a medical academic from Vanderbilt University in Nashville, Tennessee, had been moved by the sentiments in the 'Letters to No-one'. She commented that if someone is asked to write about their feelings about retirement, and share them, the results might be very different from someone describing their hopes and fears and putting them in an envelope which might never be discovered.

The first letter was dated April 1989 and a final one in October 1989, just a few weeks after retiring. In April, she described her busy life in practice as 'rushing and running' and wondered what was to be when this stopped. She worried about the patients she had cared for over the past four decades whose personal problems, even more than their strictly medical ones, affected her deeply. Focussed firmly on the present, she saw little value in celebrating retirement but contented herself that she had established a thriving medical practice, living the life of an urban Glasgow general practitioner touching the lives of many people, overwhelmed by their affection and involved in all aspects of their care.

> Is it a celebration? I have prepared myself that at the age of three score and ten I should retire. It seems now the right decision but when shall I know? All my life I have rushed and run and when the running and rushing stops, what then? This is what worries me. I am not used to sitting about but neither am I trained for anything else and physically I do not feel up to starting something new. And what of my temperament—intolerant in a word. However, my decision is resolute.

Her description of herself as 'intolerant' is interesting. She was certainly intolerant of bureaucracy and health service delays, of alcoholism and malingering, but tolerant of all she met, and her ability to care was legendary. Her strong sense of right and justice compelled her to support those who needed help but to take issue with patients who tried to abuse the system.

It was clear that her care was not just a matter of paying attention to cases in a clinic but a concern for each patient's wellbeing that persisted all through her working life. This concern was as strong at her retiral as it had been throughout her working life, as she wrote in the first letter:

> At work I am upset by the distressing stories of hardship among young and old. I have compiled several lists of names of people with problems—each of which could fill a book. What of GD his life is a nightmare—if anyone had a nightmare so bad. What of CM, age 89 whose son, a doctor, died at thirty years of age, afraid that her money will run out—what then? What of SE, unmarried with three handicapped children and can't cope.

The final concern in the first letter was about keeping up-to-date with medical developments, not to mention the frequent periods of re-organisation experienced by National Health Service primary care.

The pressures of medicine today are too great. The new and complex drugs with their interactions and side effects, one must be alert and quickly reactive. I do not think I could continue to be up to my own expected standard and target and give of my best. Although, I do think, at the moment, I am no worse than anyone else—am I being complacent?

She was also unprepared for a practice retirement event:

I did not want [a retirement gift of] a painting [but] the office staff insist. Do they think it is a celebration—my going?

If the first letter represented her thoughts about retiring some months before submitting her resignation, there is a change by the time of the second letter, in July 1989. Here, she faces the reality that retirement will bring:

The die is cast. My resignation has been tendered and a notice of my retiral has been posted. The sad part of me is that I am going and will lose contact with all those who have been part of my life for 43 years. The glad part is the emotional sentiments of my patients and friends, because that is what these people have become. I am overwhelmed that most think that I am taking early retiral although many know that I have been working in Ibrox for 43 years. . . . The over 70s are sad and some are tearful as they speak of their memories of their parents, children and grandchildren. In some families I am on my fifth generation. The over 50s say I deserve my retiral and wish me a long retiral to enjoy whatever I choose to do. The younger [ones] are also reminiscing and I am surprised at those who kiss and hope that we shall meet again. The children will miss me—perhaps my successors will be happy to display their school photographs, which they love to bring, their paintings and enjoy a little sweet which they know I keep for them in the top drawer.

In some ways, the final letter, written on the 5th of October 1989, just after finishing work and clearing her desk on the last day of September, is quite surprising given the detailed introspection which preceded it. The date of retiral was timed to lead into the preparation time for a pre-arranged holiday so that the new life would follow an overseas trip and not a regular workday. On her last day at work, there was a special retirement party which she described in the October letter as 'probably one of the outstanding days of my life: a party arranged in the surgery by the staff'. More than anything else, the emotions generated by the retirement party and the cards, messages and small gifts from many dozens of patients produced an awareness that the oral history study that I had proposed was a fitting way to perpetuate her legacy and indicate the relationships which develop over the generations of caring. She noted: 'I have officially retired and now realise that this is a fact'.

Through the words of her former patients, we will discover how these aims worked out in practice with her acceptance as a practitioner with rare skills of empathy, judgement and resilience. As a partner in a large medical practice from the summer of 1946, she had to establish herself as a trusted listener, confidant, diagnostician and practitioner. Forty-three years in one medical practice did not dim her enthusiasm for her work or for the ethos of the National Health Service which sought from the outset to give quality medicine to the entire population, free of charge at the point of contact. Her marriage and formation of a GP partnership drew together all these strands in a positive way:

> If my late husband had not been discharged from the army at that particular time, I should not have been in general practice and would have missed all this. I do not think that any branch of medicine could give the same sort of satisfaction or relationship.

In the first days in the practice, when the attention of the doctor counted for as much as the prescribed medication, there was a sense of appreciation which always remained with the patient. Mercer et al. noted that GP principals in Scotland showed continuing wide-spread support for holistic primary care and frustration at a system which appears to discourage such a priority.[24] Their study shows that the quality agenda in general practice has focussed more on access and bio-medical aspects of care than on relationship between patient and doctor. These oral history interviews show the vital importance of this relationship and gives an insight into how various factors, such as implicit trust, played out in one inner-city Glasgow practice (Figure 1.1).

In this chapter, the scene has been set for the oral history study and its analysis.

GLASGOW

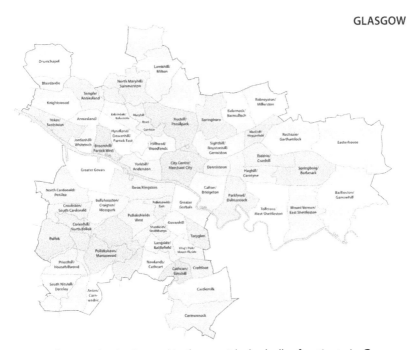

Figure 1.1 The practice is situated in Ibrox, with the bulk of patients in Govan, Cardonald and Pollok but some also as far as Darnley, Arden and Castlemilk. The Southern General Hospital is in Greater Govan, Leverndale Hospital in Pollok, the Victoria Infirmary in Battlefield with the Western Infirmary and the Royal Hospital for Sick Children in the Yorkhill area. (© vectorstock)

NOTES

1 Irvine Loudon, John Horder, and Charles Webster, *General Practice under the National Health Service 1948–1977* (Clarendon Press, Oxford, 1998). The book provides an invaluable guide to general practice in the first years of the National Health Service, but the evidence provided comes from medical practitioners or social scientists rather than patients.

2 There is an extensive literature on patient views on such issues as practice appointments and consulting a woman doctor. There is much less on oral history and general practice. Paul Thompson, a leading figure in oral history research, pointed to its value in medicine in P. Thompson, Oral History and the History of Medicine, *Social History of Medicine*, 4 (2), 1991, pp. 371–373. In 2002, the *British Journal of General Practice* printed a series of articles on oral history and general practice with Paisley GPs interviewed by a social scientist: G. Smith, M. Nicolson, and G. C. M. Watt, An Oral History of Everyday General Practice: Speaking for a Change, *British Journal of General Practice*, 52 (479), 2002, pp. 516–517; G. Smith and M. Nicolson, Re-expressing the Division of British Medicine under the NHS: The Importance of Locality in General 'Practitioners' Oral Histories, *Social Science and Medicine*, 64, 2007, pp. 938–948; G. Smith and M. Nicolson, An Oral History of General Practice 6: Beyond the Practice: The Changing Relationship with Secondary Care, *British Journal of General Practice*, 52 (484), 2002, pp. 956–957; D. Hannay, Oral History and Qualitative Research, *British Journal of General Practice*, 52 (479), 2002, p. 515.

3 Catherine Pope, Sue Ziebland and Nicholas Mays, Analysing Qualitative Data, *BMJ*, 320, 2000, p. 114. They concluded that 'High quality analysis of qualitative data depends on the skill, vision and integrity of the researcher'. Another approach uses grounded theory which was introduced by Glaser and Straus in 1967 to obviate the need to apply statistical methods to the interview data, and aspects were updated in 1991; see G. Thomas and D. James, Reinventing Grounded Theory: Some Questions About Theory, Ground and Discovery, *British Educational Research Journal*, 32 (6), 2006, pp. 767–795. Barney G. Glaser and Anselm L. Strauss, *Discovery of Grounded Theory: Strategies for Qualitative Research* (Transaction Publishers, New York, 1999) (first published in 1967). Brian D. Haig, Grounded Theory as Scientific Method, *Philosophy of Education*, 28 (1), 1995, pp. 1–11.

4 Sue Ziebland and Ann McPherson, Making Sense of Qualitative Data Analysis: An Introduction with Illustrations from DIPEx (Personal Experiences of Health and Illness), *Medical Education*, 40 (5), 2006, pp. 405–414.

5 Angela Bartie and Arthur McIvor, Oral History in Scotland, *The Scottish Historical Review*, 92 (234), 2013, Supplement: The State of Early Modern and Modern Scottish Histories, 108–136.

6 RES reference number: 07/S0701/75.

7 Letter from Professor Arthur McIvor, to Professor Jess Dawson, MD Ethics Committee, 15/6/2021.

8 Sir Ronald Gibson, *The Family Doctor: His Life and History* (London, 1981), p. 1. The book was written at a time when most family doctors were male.

9 Philip R. Myerscough, *Talking with Patients: A Basic Clinical Skill* (Oxford Medical Publications, Oxford, 1989), pp. 27–37.

10 Stewart W. Mercer, Peter G. Cawston and Annemieke P. Bikker, Quality in General Practice Consultations; A Qualitative Study of the Views of Patients

Living in an Area of High Socio-Economic Deprivation in Scotland, *BMC Family Practice*, 8, 2007, Article number: 22.
11 Stewart W. Mercer, Bhautesh D. Jani, Margaret Maxwell, Samuel Y. S. Wong, and Graham C. M. Watt, Patient Enablement Requires Physician Empathy: A Cross-Sectional Study of General Practice Consultations in Areas of High and Low Socioeconomic Deprivation in Scotland, *MC Family Practice*, 13, 2012, p. 6.
12 Valerie Yow, 'Do I Like Them Too Much?' Effects of the Oral History Interview on the Interviewer and Vice Versa, in Robert Perks and Alistair Thomson, editors, *The Oral History Reader*, pp. 54–72.
13 Andrew Carnegie (1835–1919) was born in Dunfermline but migrated to the United States with his family at the age of 12. He became the richest man in America through his steel company and prudent investments. The Scottish universities benefitted from a share of the $350 million (about $65 billion in 2022 values) he gave to charity in the last years of his life.
14 The triple qualification is Licentiate of the Royal Colleges of Physicians and Surgeons of Edinburgh and the unitary Royal College of Physicians and Surgeons in Glasgow. (LRCP&S Glasgow and LRCP and LRCS Edinburgh).
15 Carol Dyhouse, *No Distinction of Sex? Women in the British Universities 1870–1939* (UCL Press, London, 1995), p. 249. In 1920–1921, there had been 1,122 women at the University of Glasgow out of 4,518 (24.0%), and by 1934–1935, there were 1,149 women out of 4,390 (26.1%). Figures from *Returns of the University Grants Committee*.
16 Writing on behalf of the London Association of the Medical Women's Federation, F Lefford noted that equality of access to medical courses had not led to equality of access of employment. See F. Lefford, Prejudice against Women Doctors, *British Medical Journal (Clinical Research Edition)*, 294 (6575), 1987, p. 838.
17 Letter on file with author.
18 Ibid.
19 Ibid.
20 Wendy Alexander, *First Ladies of Medicine* (University of Glasgow, Glasgow, 1987), p. 49.
21 E. Moberley Bell, *Storming the Citadel: The Rise of the Woman Doctor* (Constable, London, 1953), p. 171.
22 Obituary of Albert Sharman DSc PhD MD FRCS (Glas) FRCOG, *BMJ*, 1970, p. 634.
23 The average practice list size (per doctor) was 2,206 in Scotland in 1951. Quoted in Anne Digby, *The Evolution of British General Practice 1850–1948* (Oxford University Press, Oxford, 1999), p. 336.
24 Harutomo Hasegawa, David Reilly, Stewart W. Mercer, and Annemieke P. Bikker, Holism in Primary Care: The Views of Scotland's General Practitioners, *Primary Health Care Research and Development*, 6 (4), 2006, pp. 320–328. https://doi.org/10.1191/1463423605pc248oa. Published online by Cambridge University Press: 31 October 2006.

2

The Medical Background

WOMEN IN MEDICINE

Dr Ockrim had seen her destiny in medicine from an early stage. In later life, she would recount stories of her medical heroines who had entered the previously closed male medical world just a generation before her birth. These women graduates were well aware of the sentiments expressed sixty years earlier by Edith Pechey in a lecture at the London School of Medicine for Women in 1882:

> We were to understand that no one would wish to consult us unless we were the best doctors to be had in our neighbourhood, so she said that we were to see that we were.

Women like Sophia Jex-Blake (1840–1912) and Elizabeth Garrett Anderson (1836–1917) had always had a warm place in her heart, and their lengthy struggle, with many setbacks, for acceptance in Britain was one of which she was immensely proud.[1] Sophia Jex-Blake was in America in 1867 trying hard, but unsuccessfully, to enter Harvard University. She moved on to New York for some private teaching in anatomy after having had some informal clinical experience at the Massachusetts General Hospital.[2] Undaunted, Jex-Blake returned first to medical studies in Edinburgh and then to London, where she became the leader of the movement for women's medical studies, founding the London Medical School for Women in 1874. Elizabeth Garrett Anderson finally obtained a licence (LSA) in 1865 from the Society of Apothecaries to practise medicine, the first woman qualified in Britain to do so openly. She had been refused entry to more regular places of medical studies but obtained her qualifications through a loophole in the Society's regulations.

Some of the first women doctors had started their medical training by enrolling in a nursing course. Women could argue that nurses had proved themselves well able to act in situations from which male doctors wished to exclude their female counterparts.[3] However, it was the feeling of aspiring middle-class women doctors that nursing represented a type of work they did not wish to undertake. Sophia Jex-Blake had asked, in 1872, why women should be as follows:

> be limited to merely the mechanical details and wearisome routine of nursing, while to men is reserved all intelligent knowledge of disease?[4]

DOI: 10.1201/9781003369301-2

We have seen that another heroine was Elsie Inglis, who completed her training at the Glasgow Royal Infirmary, as Dr Ockrim was to do some fifty years later.[5] Inglis opened a maternity hospital in Edinburgh in 1894, named The Hospice, for poor women alongside a midwifery resource and training centre. This was the forerunner of the Elsie Inglis Memorial Hospital, where Dr Ockrim worked after leaving the Glasgow Royal Infirmary in 1943 and which operated as a maternity until closed by the NHS in 1988.

In the first decades of the twentieth century, there was a continuing reluctance to employ women if qualified men were available, and marriage was often seen as a bar to establish a medical career. While the first medical women had proved their worth in military hospitals during World War I, the post-war period still posed difficulties for women seeking a medical career.[6] Even before World War I, about a quarter of women graduates opted for a career in general practice which seemed to offer a better working option.[7] As late as the 1930s, medical women working for the Glasgow Corporation had to resign from their positions on marriage.[8] Even though more than thirty years had passed since the establishment of the women's medical school in Glasgow, their presence was still regarded as being in 'the experimental stage', and there was still the general feeling that bringing too much public attention to the question could be counterproductive.[9]

Medical studies for women began in the University of Glasgow with the opening of the doors of Queen Margaret College in Glasgow in 1890. This gave women in the West of Scotland the opportunity to study and graduate in medicine through their own medical school. Glasgow was, therefore, in fourth place in Britain in providing facilities for women to study medicine. Within a few years, women were allowed to matriculate at Glasgow University, though the separate lectures continued.[10] There were still many attitudes to be changed, but by the time Dr Ockrim was born, in 1919, there were around 1,500 women on the medical register in Britain, and even within Glasgow's mainly immigrant Jewish community, the first few women doctors had already qualified.

Though the problems of admission to the medical register had been solved by the time that Dr Ockrim was leaving school in 1938, there was still no equality of opportunity for female medical graduates in Glasgow's main voluntary hospitals.[11] The Royal Infirmary, where she held a surgical residency post in 1943, had been open to women since 1899. In contrast, the Western Infirmary only began to employ women residents during World War II, owing to the reduced number of young male doctors because of the number of call-ups to the army. Women were also not admitted to residency posts at the Victoria Infirmary.

While female doctors had to struggle to assert their right to a university education, there was a common attitude in the community that shared the view that 'learning was for the men'. One oral history participant described how she had worked and saved to give her daughter the education and career she had been denied, even though her family had not approved:

I never had the chance of getting an education. You were always told that it was men that got educated, not women. . . . I went and done cleaning to gather up money to put her through that. She was doing that cancer and leukaemia [research] . . . she had a mind of her own and I wasn't standing in her way, because I never got a chance.

(DMc)

I have shown how the Scottish medical schools had been open almost from the first to Jewish medical students, and when Dr Ockrim began her studies at Glasgow University in 1938, there were hundreds of American Jewish medical students, excluded by a quota system from studying in the United States, studying medicine in Scotland. At the same time, from 1933 onwards, there had been hundreds of mainly Jewish doctors, refugees from Nazism, requalifying in Scotland. There was no problem for Jewish students entering medical studies in Scotland, although some prestigious medical appointments in the main teaching hospitals were closed to Jews until more recent times.[12]

The medical undergraduate curriculum in the 1940s did not include any experience of general practice, though any graduate would be aware of the opportunities offered by the ability to set up in practice with a relatively modest outlay and no need to have any further post-graduate training. Many of the women entering general practice had a medical family background which facilitated entry to otherwise male-dominated practices. Women also had the advantage that they were often seen as 'guides and wise counsellors in all that concerns the physical welfare of the family'.[13]

Anne Digby, writing in 1999, noted that general practice for women had changed little in the previous seventy years, comprising mainly paediatrics, obstetrics and gynaecology, birth-control advice and what was described as 'female neurosis'.[14] She remarked that medical women gravitated to general practice where their skills were appreciated and where they developed a greater personal closeness that was more rarely found (or at least acknowledged) amongst their male colleagues.[15]

In her historical study of gender issues in medicine and science in Scotland over the past 300 years, Yeo noted that, in the usual historiography, with the exception of midwifery training, shared with male medical students in Edinburgh, Aberdeen and Glasgow, women have been pushed to the margins of modernity, as traditional healers in the countryside and in the private sphere of the family.[16] While women were facing difficulties with advancement in the medical profession in the early twentieth century, they established a near-monopoly over a range of other health professions, including nursing, health visiting and midwifery. The national health crisis, exemplified by the poor physical health of army recruits in the Boer War, led to the *Report of the Interdepartmental Committee on Physical Deterioration*. This put the health, especially of mothers and children, at the centre of the national agenda. As Yeo notes, the debate was overlaid with concern for the welfare of the Empire and with eugenic issues affecting the British race. The concern led inexorably to the gradual development of the welfare state in subsequent decades.

With the increased presence of women in general practice following World War II, a number of studies have examined the implications for general practice, with concerns that a female preference for part-time working, usually because of family commitments, would lead to a fall in the numbers of general practitioners available to treat patients.[17] McKinstry asked in 2008, 'Are there too many female medical graduates?'[18] The answer he gave was 'yes', pointing to the women doctors who chose to work part-time early in their careers for child-care, opting to continue with part-time working when their children became independent. Though acknowledging that, for years, women have been unfairly discriminated against in medicine, McKinstry proclaimed the need for full equality of opportunity but maintained that there was a need:

> in the absence of a profound change in our society in terms of responsibility for child-care, we need to take a balanced approach to recruitment in the interests of both equity and future delivery of services.

An important component of general practice was the management of pregnancy and childbirth. However, the relationship between women doctors and midwives was complex. The development of midwifery as a professional discipline had led to anxiety within the male medical profession who recognised the need for better care of routine pregnancies, especially amongst the poor, but found it hard to cope with a better educated midwife.[19] However, in practice, midwifery remained confined to older, part-time and often working-class women rather being seen as an alternative to a medical career. In contrast, a subject like obstetrics and gynaecology involved years of gaining clinical experience followed by specialist examinations.

It was the Goodenough Report of 1944, which was implemented after World War II, which made Exchequer Grants to medical schools conditional on their being co-educational.[20] The report also recommended that hospital appointments should now be open to men and women on equal terms. While prejudice against women in medicine undoubtedly persisted well into the twentieth century, Dingwall points out that those seeking professional careers for women in the pre–World War II era were a minority and certainly did not represent a mass movement.[21] In the case of medicine, she notes that women were seeking to enter a profession that was both intellectual and practical and that often it was the 'reticence and prescriptive code of middle class behaviour' to be found amongst women as well as men that caused the difficulties especially at examinations.[22]

Entering a predominantly working-class practice in 1946, Dr Ockrim must have realised that having a woman doctor as an equal partner in the practice would take some time for acceptance. At the same time, Dr Ockrim was determined to have a career, a marriage and a family at a time when less than a third of female medical graduates were working full-time.[23] Even as late as 1987, it was still being said that equality of access to medical schools had not led to equality of access to senior hospital appointments, leaving women behind in more junior positions.[24]

The current age, when women now outnumber men in British medical schools, was a world away from the era when Dr Ockrim graduated. In 1943, the women who graduated with her were still a clear minority. They had only recently been included in the graduation booklet, produced annually by the graduates themselves with photographs and quotes about staff and students. That this was a concession was illustrated by the placement of the new women doctors in a group at the back of the booklet. With many male doctors being called up for military service during World War II, their places were often filled by recent retirees rather than underemployed women doctors.[25] Dr Ockrim had showed perseverance in her studies and medical work, but she would still encounter patients who were reluctant to consult a female doctor.

Consulting a Woman Doctor

There have been many studies which look at the preferences that patients have when choosing their doctor. Questions are often asked about age, ethnic background, place of qualification as well as gender. One such study looked at patient preferences both for hospital doctors and general practitioners looking at just these questions.[26] In 1967, Hopkin and colleagues felt that the issue was 'probably marginal' as they 'seldom encounter any overt difficulty as to whether a man or a woman attends a patient'.[27] However, more detailed studies in recent decades have produced a more nuanced picture. As might be expected, given patient contacts with GPs often lasting for many decades, results showed that people were more specific about selecting GPs than hospital consultants, and they also showed a preference for UK-trained doctors.

Sally Nichols conducted a postal survey of 512 women in 1987, looking at women's preferences for the sex of a doctor.[28] Less than one in ten said they would prefer to see a female general practitioner for general health problems, compared with nearly six out of ten for women's health problems. Similarly, almost 60% would prefer to see a female health professional for cervical screening and for breast screening by physical examination and instruction in self-examination. She concluded that more women general practitioners might increase compliance rates for cervical screening among high-risk groups. Thus, for sexual issues or intimate examinations, women seek a female doctor and male patients favour a male doctor.[29]

Studies have shown that women doctors saw considerably more women with women's health problems than did their male colleagues.[30] Women were more likely to consult a woman general practitioner if she was more available, and younger women were more likely than older women to choose female general practitioners. Many studies also show that women general practitioners had longer consultations than their male colleagues for a variety of reasons based on the style of practice but mainly because more health problems were presented per consultation.[31] Women often engaged more in preventive services and were felt to have a more supportive manner.

Weisman and Teitelbaum considered that physician gender might impact mainly on the relationship through patients' different expectations of male and female physicians, pointing out that patients may seek a doctor of the same gender as a key factor promoting a better communication of information, establishing a climate of rapport and facilitating negotiation.[32] These last issues are important in motivating patients over an extended period.

Waller found that women are important users of health care services, attending their general practitioner more frequently than men and receiving more prescribed drugs.[33] She showed that women patients believe women doctors to have the good qualities of both male and female physicians, like assertiveness and initiative but also tenderness and nurturance, and pointed to evidence that women doctors give their female patients more surgery time than is allocated to them by male doctors. In practices where there were no women doctors, about half of women attending stated that they wanted to see a female GP in at least some circumstances.[34] Plunkett and colleagues studied the effects of gender in selecting an obstetrician or a gynaecologist.[35] Of those women who expressed a preference, most favoured female doctors, but when asked to consider this preference in relation to experience, bedside manner and competency, gender became a much less salient consideration.

In brief, the studies showed that patients prefer to see doctors similar to them in terms of ethnicity and gender, especially when dealing with more intimate health problems. For practices with a significant presence of Asian patients, the issues of female reluctance, especially for Pakistani women, to be examined by a male doctor arise.[36] The recent rise in the proportion of women entering medicine has not ended gender prejudice, though women in medicine have made significant progress in recent decades.

DEPRIVATION IN GLASGOW AND ITS HEALTH CONSEQUENCES: THE GLASGOW EFFECT

One of the leading figures in understanding general practice and developing its research-based underpinning was Julian Tudor Hart (1927–2018), who described what he called the Inverse Care Law, which applied to areas of socio-economic deprivation.[37] He noted this:

> the availability of good medical care tends to vary inversely with the need for it in the population served. In areas with most sickness and death, general practitioners have more work, larger lists, less hospital support, and inherit more clinically ineffective traditions of consultation, than in the healthiest areas.

Tudor Hart's perceptive analysis of health care in deprived areas applied especially in cities like Glasgow. Taking a Glasgow working-class practice, near to docks and shipyards, inevitably brought its share of exposure to a wide range of diseases and to multiple pathologies. The classic undergraduate teaching was that the cause of the symptoms of younger patients would be a single pathology, while in older patients, multiple illnesses could co-exist. This was clearly not how it seemed to be in real life, as recent studies have indicated that, especially in Scottish practices with a high level of deprivation, multiple pathologies, including problems with mental health, could exist in younger patients, too, causing both an increase in general practitioner workload and emphasising the importance of good continuing care.

This aspect of primary care features strongly in this study. It is centred in an area of Glasgow which has experienced many decades of health and social problems, placing stresses on the doctors and the nurses, health visitors and social workers serving this community. In areas like Ibrox and Govan, consultation rates and demands for house calls were high, and the patients often experienced a range of health and social problems requiring a solution or at least amelioration within a tight consulting time scale. It was said that experts would come to Glasgow to study its notoriety in the field of health and health care and were 'prepared to be shocked. They have been rarely disappointed'.[38] Glasgow's health has long been notorious. One of the first to comment on the health of Glasgow's poor was Friedrich Engels, on his visit to Glasgow in 1844, who commented that he 'did not believe, until [he] visited the wynds of Glasgow, that so large an amount of filth, crime, misery and disease existed in one spot in any civilized country'.[39]

Research has confirmed the persistence of a Glasgow Effect.[40] Liverpool and Manchester have similar levels of deprivation, but Glasgow continues to experience levels of poor health 'over and above that explained by socio-economic circumstances'. Walsh et al. considered reasons for this excess morbidity and considered that Glasgow was more vulnerable than other cities, such as Liverpool and Manchester, because of historic deprivation, loss of heavy industries, overcrowding and adverse social policies.[41]

In their detailed statistical analysis of Scotland's health parameters, produced in 1991, at the time the interviews were conducted, Carstairs and Morris painted a depressing picture of Scotland's health inequalities.[42] They used population information obtained from census returns to lay bare the close link between socio-economic factors and health. They showed how health inequalities between richest and poorest areas started with the risks associated with birth and continued through life with 'the gradients in mortality being steepest in younger adults but nevertheless continuing into older ages'.[43]

Glasgow had by far the highest number in the most socially and economically deprived categories at 50%—no other area in Scotland even came close.[44] The core area of the practice, G51, was divided into four sub-areas in the study. Two were in category seven, the most deprived, and two in category six. G51 1, which is where the surgery is situated, was in category six, and some of the areas where slum clearance households were resettled, such as G53, showed a similar level of deprivation to G51. They showed that there was a substantial excess of multimorbidity in young and middle-aged adults living in the most deprived areas. These adults had the same prevalence of multiple morbidities as people aged about 10–15 years older living in the most affluent areas. Further, it showed that women had higher rates of multimorbidity than did men and consistently higher rates of mental health disorders.[45] In 2012, a large group of general practitioners working in the most deprived areas of Scotland, described as the 'Deep End', came together to share experiences and views on providing best quality health care to their vulnerable populations.[46]

The NHS began by absorbing the buildings and structures which had served the local populations in earlier decades. In many cases, this carried a stigma which it took many years to overcome. The main hospital provision in the practice area was supplied by the Southern General Hospital. It was originally known as the Govan Combination Poorhouse and was built on the Merryflats Estate to replace previous poorhouse buildings nearby.[47] There was a poorhouse, an asylum building to the south and a further building to the north. The complex was renamed the Southern General Hospital in 1923, and the last of the poorhouse beds disappeared in 1936. However, the psychogeriatric wards had changed little by the time I started postgraduation work at the hospital in 1972.

The poor were not required to be housed in poorhouses, as in England, but could be given relief in cash or kind.[48] Many poorhouses were built, however, and in the cities, parishes often joined together to build one. The poorhouses were intended for the sick and destitute poor, and inmates were segregated into male and female areas, and this segregation continued into differentiating between the deserving and non-deserving poor. These buildings catered extensively to those suffering from mental illness and provided very basic accommodation though with asylum and infirmary beds.[49]

The practice, too, had to consider the provision of its own premises. By 1986, it was realised that the increasingly cramped tenement flat in Cessnock Street was no longer 'fit for purpose'. At the same time, the building was due to be renovated by the City's Housing Department, and there was to be no room for a doctors' surgery. The uncomfortable last months in an otherwise empty and vandalised building will be discussed later. The search began to find alternative premises, and fortunately, a site, also belonging to the City of Glasgow, was identified just three streets away. It was at the edge of a proposed sheltered housing development whose building was yet to start. The site had previously belonged to a timber yard, as the ground had not been thought to be suitable for tenement construction a century before, due to the presence of some underground quarrying. With new building techniques and a more modest building planned, the 1,200-square-metre site was cleared for construction.

The existence of the General Practice Finance Corporation (GPFC), established under the GP Charter of 1965, revolutionised the funding for practices, enabling suitable premises from which better levels of care could be delivered. In addition, the cost rent and notional rent schemes offered by the NHS made financing the building of a new purpose-built facility entirely practical. Cost rent reimbursed practices for borrowing funds for practice premises, while notional rent made provision for enhanced payment when inflation took the cost of renting similar premises above the cost-rent level.[50] Without the approvals required for GPFC funding, the project would never have succeeded. GPFC terms and conditions were closely aligned with National Health Service regulations and provided the needed incentive for improving general practice facilities.

WHAT THE VOICES TELL US

It was Marshall Marinker, Professor of Community Health, University of Leicester, who taught GPs to think about the care they provide and the relationship with their patients in new and challenging ways.[51] He pointed to the changing way in which the patient's problem, or illness, came to be understood by the doctor. He considered that this was because general practitioners had developed the self-confidence to challenge the biomedical model taught at university which did not always help with the problems posed by their patients.[52]

Doctors see people at their most vulnerable. They offer an account of their symptoms to their physician and accept a loss of personal autonomy as they trust that the therapeutic process, in whatever form it follows, will be to their benefit. Marinker urges practitioners to be aware 'of the power not only for good but also for evil, in the clinical transaction'. Marinker described how the patient presents his disorganised story which the doctor sorts and shapes this presentation to make a diagnosis for the patient.

Marinker saw Balint as the leading figure in establishing an understanding of the doctor–patient relationship and understanding how the physician's persona becomes part of the therapeutic process.[53] From this starting point, Marinker divided ill-health into three categories: disease (diagnosis), sickness (what other people see) and illness (what the patient feels), indicating that becoming a patient involves forming a healing relationship with a doctor or other health care professionals. Marinker conducted a study with Balint and other colleagues in 1970, looking at patients who were receiving a repeat prescription for medication often over a period of many years.[54] They found that before the repeat prescription started, the patient had reported illness which despite investigation had not yielded a diagnosis. Once the repeat prescription began, 'the doctor-patient relationship became peaceful, and the patient seemed to function more or less effectively in his own environment'. Marinker concluded as follows:

> the patient had no demonstrable disease, he no longer complained of an illness, and he rarely seemed to occupy the role and status of sick person. The act of consulting, the giving and receiving of the prescription, seemed to constitute its own reason.

In another paper looking at compliance with long-term medication required to prevent serious illness, he discovered that non-compliance was no more deviant than compliant, finding that members of a medical working group on compliance admitted that that they rarely took medication as prescribed. He quoted Franz Kafka: 'To write prescriptions is easy, but to come to an understanding of people is hard'.[55]

Marinker claimed that 'there is a paradox at the root of modern medicine'.[56] He indicated that 'clinical method is concerned to compare the reality of the unique individual with the model of the ideal disease'. The benefits of this approach have led to major advances in modern medicine and behavioural science. At the same time, doctors have to understand the patient, his experiences, beliefs and background. By 1990, with further NHS reorganisation, he noted that 'the tasks of the intimate consultation between doctor and patient were being disaggregated and shared with others'.[57]

Between the publication of Balint's *The Doctor, His Patient and the Illness* in 1957 and the Royal College of General Practitioners' *The Future General Practitioner* in 1972, Ian McWhinney published a key paper on the emerging topic of family medicine as an academic discipline.[58] McWhinney based this topic on general practice constituting a unique field of action, a defined body of knowledge, an active area of research and a training which is intellectually rigorous. Iona Heath has argued for a rebalancing of the two sides in every clinical consultation, acknowledging that there are situations 'for which evidence-based medicine has no answers' and that trying 'to describe people in terms of data from biomedical science . . . are not, and will never be, enough'.[59] She acknowledges that evidence-based medicine provides doctors with 'an alphabet—but, as clinicians, we remain unsure of the language'. This study shows how oral history can provide that language.

One theme which formed a significant party of collective memories is related to stigma. We will see how stigma operated in many other aspects of patient care. It was seen in many illnesses, especially related to tuberculosis and mental health issues, and we can see how stigma affected patients and families in later chapters. Social science research on stigma has grown dramatically over the past two decades. Link and Phelan note this:

> because there are so many stigmatized circumstances and because stigmatizing processes can affect multiple domains of people's lives, stigmatization probably has a dramatic bearing on the distribution of life chances in such areas as earnings, housing, criminal involvement, health, and life itself.[60]

Stigma, therefore, calls into question a person's moral character and choices, and their right to full membership in society. Thus, feelings of stigma can influence behaviour, create anxiety, reduce interaction with other people and compromise recovery prospects. In the interviews, we encounter memories of means-tested benefits, social welfare provision of inferior housing, and paternalistic and parsimonious provision of children's clothing and other items remain fresh. Some stigmas are related to health, tuberculosis, psychiatric illnesses and physical deformities, for example, and some to behaviour which falls outside society norms, like addiction and homosexuality, and finally, being a member of a group, nationality, religion or race, which is seen as 'different'.[61]

HISTORY OF THE PRACTICE

When these interviews were carried out, the founder of the practice, Dr Stevan George, had left Glasgow more than forty years earlier. Nevertheless, these recollections indicate a great deal of affection and acceptance for the abilities and personality of the young man who had come to Scotland as a refugee during World War I. Stevan George (1900–1967) was born Slavko Djordjević in Serbia.[62] Stevan George had arrived in Glasgow in 1916, one of the Serbian boys, aged between 12 and 17, who had survived what is known as the Retreat—a perilous journey over the mountains of Albania and Montenegro during the winter to escape capture after their country suffered catastrophic defeat at the hands of Germany and its allies.[63] He finished his school studies at Hillhead High School then studied medicine at the University of Glasgow, where he won a rugby blue.

George graduated in 1924, and after marriage, he set up his own practice in Blackburn Street in the Kinning Park area of Glasgow as a general practitioner. Setting up alone in a practice meant a period of uncertainty while recruiting patients through the National Health Insurance (NHI) scheme or through funding from members of trade unions or friendly societies.[64] The NHI was set up by the National Insurance Act of 1911, creating a system of health cover for industrial workers in Great Britain based on contributions from employers, the government and the workers themselves. The alternative to a single-handed practice would have been to join an existing practice as an assistant, who might have the opportunity for partnership at some unspecified time in the future or to become a junior partner, fully sharing the workload but receiving a far lower income than the senior partner.[65]

Digby notes that many partnerships foundered because of different approaches to practice procedures, especially related to income or attitudes to doctors from different backgrounds, whether religious or ethnic. By setting up his own practice, George could make his own decisions, be responsible for his patients and keep the practice profits for himself. After he opened his surgery in Blackburn Street, he began to enlist local support and to impress potential patients not just with his skills but also with his personality. The National Insurance Act had made the income of general practitioners more secure, and it was a straightforward procedure to set up a new and independent practice, as the establishment of the doctor's panel gave both patient and doctor an improved framework for care.[66] The NHI, as it was known, had provided only for a basic level of medical services. Income was mainly derived from capitation fees, so there was little incentive by many GPs to provide anything beyond basic services. After 1948, the practice workload increased significantly as NHS provision extended the range of what was available.[67]

Around 1929, he moved to more spacious accommodation a few hundred yards along Paisley Road West at 2 Cessnock Street, which allowed him and his growing family to live 'on the job'.[68] This gave him the room to employ an assistant doctor. He later moved from Cessnock Street and brought in a resident caretaker to look after the premises. The surgery area began with two good-sized consulting rooms, with running water and examination couches which could be screened off, and there was a very small reception area that housed the patients' notes.[69]

There was a feeling that he should have been recognised for his work during the Clydeside Blitz when he treated severely injured patients amongst the rubble of bombed-out buildings. The local damage in the practice area was considerable. However, he never received an award.

By this time, it was coming up for war and he did wonderful work—and tunnelled and saved people and gave them morphine injections and was—his name was put forward for the George Medal—he refused it. He turned it down for the very simple reason—he was one of a few who had done practically the same as what he was doing.

(V&IT)

Dr George got the George Medal for that, because he crawled under all that debris. He, and my father and my father's mate. He had to administer the painkilling drugs to the people under there.

(DR)

Some of the older patients recalled Stevan George and his role in the practice and had their own recollections of his arrival in the practice, different in some details from the official record.

There was a lot of people in that church with a bit of money. They had a very strong foreign mission. . . . There was two ladies who were the leading lights in this foreign mission and they went to Yugoslavia, and it was probably a similar situation as just now, and they brought back this young Serbian with them, and to my knowledge they helped him and got him through university and that's actually how he came to be in Britain.

(IL)

Memories of the first surgery indicated it was very basic, recalled as follows:

I think it was a small room at the top of Blackburn Street. Wooden forms to sit on. Very small. [The consulting room was] even smaller. Just the leather couch. Then it went to Cessnock.

(HT)

He was just there on his own, most of the time, and it was like one big waiting room where you all sat in a circle and kept moving on as it was your turn. He would shout 'Next!' for you to go in. The man was too busy to go in and out when he was alone.

(IL)

An interviewee who would have been an older teenager when Dr George left the country, remembered the following:

I suppose as a young boy my mother would take me in, and you sat in the hallway waiting for your turn to come. There was Dr George himself, but he had an assistant at one time. She was a lady doctor. The entrenched thought of people those days, nobody wanted to go to the lady doctor and there was always a big queue for Dr George.

(FC)

Yes, I remember him. He was dark—he looked Jewish. . . . Very . . . very thick eyebrows and he had the pleasant face. He had quite a heavy jowl, but he was a nice man, but he drank too much.

(IN)

I don't think I ever needed much in examinations, he would just listen to you and maybe sound your back, but nothing very thorough.

(SN)

The basic format for recording patient details was the so-called Lloyd George envelopes, into which all medical information about the patient was placed. Lloyd George had been Chancellor of the Exchequer when National Health Insurance began in 1911, and the name for the envelopes stuck. These envelopes, like the card for recording notes of consultations, were made of stiff paper, and the small size of the envelopes, which were only 5″ by 7″ gave little room for the accumulation of hospital correspondence and blood test results over the following years. In many cases, the small amount of space available for note-taking meant that even in larger practices, notes were at a minimum.[70] In a single-handed practice, notes could be very rudimentary, if they existed at all, as the doctor might keep the details of consultations in his head. Details might be summarised in just a word or two. As records became more detailed and hospital interventions more common, the envelopes became overloaded, and the practice abandoned them in 1980 in favour of A4 folders.

It seems that Stevan George's records were unbelievable—they just didn't exist.

(VK)

Stevan George had some remedies of his own. In the days before almost all medications were supplied by giant pharmaceutical companies in pre-packed containers, many local pharmacies made up preparations based on the individual recipes prescribed by the patient's doctor. One such remedy, for stomach ulcers, was called the 'six ingredients'. Most of the contents were antacids of one kind or another, but the final item was a strong dose of phenobarbitone. In the 1930s, and indeed for many decades afterwards, there was no effective way of reducing stomach acid, apart from prolonged bedrest or gastric surgery. The remedy proved to be very popular, but once the phenobarbitone was removed, it immediately fell out of favour. Another remedy showed an enquiring mind:

Dr George, at this point, asked my father would he mind if he did an experimentation on me, because he had a theory about—like fighting fire with fire, to kill the disease [asthma] by treating it with the disease sort of style. What happened was, twelve samples of sputum went into a little vial, and he took it away and brought it back in—He injected it back into me, in twelve injections. It was the District Nurse who came to do that. It was over twelve weeks—one every week.

(DR)

Many participants recalled the struggle to find the money to pay for a consultation before the NHS began:

In those days you had to be pretty bad before you saw the doctor. Well, doctors were paid. We were able to pay but families always had an aunt or somebody like that who was good with poultices. There was always some expert, and it was surprising how beneficial they were. People didn't go to the doctor if they could avoid it.

(YI)

I can recall my mother talking to another woman and there was fear in their voices because they couldn't afford a doctor. . . . The charge was six pence.

(CN)

I remember you had to pay. I remember when I was in the Victoria and Phillipshill for 6 months. My mother had to pay—I've still got it yet—7/6 for an ambulance. I've still got the receipt. You had to pay for your ambulances forby[71] your medicines and things.

(LNf)

Well, I had an uncle who was active in the Rechabites[72] and we joined the friendly society and you paid so much. If you were going into hospital, you had what they called the subscribers line. . . . The people who were contributing to these societies got this line.

(GD)

Many patients recalled the days when an alternative to the expense of consulting the doctor was to draw on the expertise of family members, friends or neighbours who were experienced in the use of folk, or popular, remedies. There was, of course, some mystique in the use of poultices or tonics and their healing properties which was thought to draw the ailment from the body. These were normally made of bread or bran as absorbents but also contained mustard and medicinal herbs and were applied directly to the body often after warming. One patient (IS) recalled that around 1940, her younger daughter was admitted to hospital with measles and that '[at that time] they just poulticed them'. Another participant described the use of the poultice as an alternative to the expense of consulting the GP:

But she burned one of us at one time. . . . Well, as I say she had her own ways for different things. Epsom salts. The poultice was the thing—kaolin and mustard poultice was the favourite then.

(DD)

I remember my mother had to pay 4/6 for the doctor and if you couldnae afford that, that was too bad. You couldnae get a doctor, so maybe you just applied to the, what they called, Parish. You had to go down to what they called the Parish, down at Summertown Road. You had to apply.

(DD)

WJ said that because of his work, there 'was an understanding that Dr Collins and I had. When I got ill, I had to be made better fast. He used to do everything he could'. YI agreed that pre-NHS, 'a whole lot of doctoring was done by the people themselves' and as follows:

Although, medication in these days—there was an awful lot of psychology about it. Doctors—their strong point was their bedside manner. I remember as a small boy, when one of the doctors would come to me if I had the 'flu. We were very impressed if they would sit there and talk to you and then you ended up with a bottle of some kind, which had great properties, according to the doctor, and it made you better.

Later during the war, Stevan George registered as a navy surgeon and was on the Queen Mary and Queen Elizabeth which transported troops across the Atlantic. The trips were hazardous due to German submarines, and he received the Atlantic Star medal. Dr George worked for some years after the war as a ship's surgeon on luxury cruise liners before settling in the Bahamas working with the medical service that extended health care to inhabitants of outlying islands. He eventually received recognition from the Crown when the Queen personally appointed him Officer of the Order of the British Empire (OBE) in 1966 at Government House in Nassau. George died the following year, just 67 years old.

Stevan George's Govan and Ibrox of the 1930s and 1940s were, in many ways, examples of local self-help and communal adhesiveness that has, to a great extent, been lost in recent decades. It may have been difficult for children to do homework in a crowded flat, but with grandparents nearby, there was room to escape. Sanitary facilities were often primitive. At the same time, there remained considerable nostalgia for the cramped tenement buildings. One study participant remembered the following:

> In the old tenements, you all had the same key to open every door and if you came home from school and your parents weren't in, you went into the neighbours. and they gave you a sandwich or a cup of tea or something till they came in. When you went into the big scheme, it was a lot different because you didn't go into each other's houses. Everyone seemed to keep themselves to themselves. In the tenements it was marvellous.
>
> (HN)

There was a period of slum clearance and intensive house building through the 1950s and 1960s. Some patients moved nearby to high-rise flats in the area. Others were rehoused further afield, and this led to depopulation of the area around the surgery. Patients who were now in peripheral areas of South-West Glasgow, like Pollok, Darnley, Nitshill and Arden, tended to stay with the practice, places that were, for the most part, considered to be part of the practice area. A few who had been rehoused in Castlemilk in South-East Glasgow and were prepared to travel to Cessnock Street also remained, though the time taken for house calls was later to cause problems, as we shall see.

> A lot of families are scattered now. They go into these big sprawling schemes. There's no community spirit or life. Of course, maybe the poverty in thae days—poverty drove people together. When I look back now. At the time I never gave it much thought, but when I look back now—it's sad. I wouldnae like to see thae days coming back again, no way.
>
> (ID)

> Oh, we were very happy, and you never needed to lock your door.
>
> (QD)

Many of the recollections of those interviewed were memories of the difficult social conditions of the past—poor housing with no indoor baths or toilets and with medical access for many conducted by schemes which related to old Poor Law provision or which came at a level of expense that caused hardship. Sanitary facilities were often shared, and conditions were poor. This could be a factor in having patients admitted to hospital.

> Just a room and kitchen. An outside toilet. I shudder to think. . . . There were four families on the landing. You just had to use the baths in Plantation St or Scotland St in Govan. . . . We had the usual wash facilities—just the big sink. I often wonder how anyone managed in thae days.
>
> (CT)

We had a [toilet on the] landing and [it was shared by] three neighbours. Oh, they would tin bath every Friday night. It was in front of the fire.

(LN)

In this chapter, the key topics of women in medicine and consulting a female doctor have been considered. Dr Ockrim was prepared to challenge existing prejudices and establish herself, her views and concern to let people follow their dreams. While a young woman (DM) who had been abused at home could tell her that 'There was something powerful about you that I liked', she quickly added that 'There was a lot of people didnae like you. I used to say to people, she's straightforward and she'll tell you to your face what she thinks'.

The practice origins explain much of what followed in terms of health care. This features in the story of the practice founder, Dr Stevan George, a refugee from Serbia and a Glasgow medical graduate, and Glasgow's unenviable reputation for social and economic deprivation which impacted on its health profile, which came to be known as the Glasgow Effect. Stevan George had made up his mind to leave Glasgow before the start of the National Health Service, when he would still be able to sell his practice.

NOTES

1 There is an extensive literature on the first women in medicine. Eileen Crofton's *A Painful Inch to Gain: Personal Experiences of Early Women Medical Students in Britain* (Fastprint Publishing, Peterborough, 2013) recounts the early history of women in medicine in Britain. Coincidentally, she graduated in medicine in the same year as Dr Ockrim (1943). See also E. Moberley Bell, *Storming the Citadel*.

2 Mary Roth Walsh, *Doctors Wanted: No Women Need Apply: Sexual Barriers in the Medical Profession 1835–1975* (New Haven, 1977), pp. 100–102.

3 For a detailed account of the history of the relationship between nurses and the first women in medicine, see Vanessa Heggie, Women Doctors and Lady Nurses: Class, Education, and the Professional Victorian Woman, *Bulletin of the History of Medicine*, 89 (2), 2015, pp. 267–292.

4 Sophia Jex-Blake, *Medical Women: Two Essays* (William Oliphant, Edinburgh, 1872), p. 8 (quoted in Vanessa Heggie, note 3, above).

5 E. Moberley Bell, *Storming the Citadel*, pp. 148–159; Hamish McPherson, Greatest Scot? The Many Talents of Elsie Inglis, *The National (Daily Newspaper of NewsQuest Media Group)*, 20 May 2020.

6 Carol Dyhouse, Driving Ambitions: Women in Pursuit of a Medical Education, 1890–1939, *Women's History Review*, 7 (3), 1998, pp. 321–343.

7 Wendy Alexander, *First Ladies of Medicine* (University of Glasgow, 1987), p. 49.

8 Comment in the *Glasgow Herald* noted by Anne Digby, *The Evolution of British General Practice*, pp. 168–169.

9 Carol Dyhouse, *No Distinction of Sex*, p. 242.

10 Johanna Geyer-Kordesch Rona Ferguson, *Blue Stockings, Black Gowns, White Coats: A Brief History of Women Entering the Medical Profession in Scotland in Celebration of One Hundred Years of Women Graduates at the University of Glasgow* (University of Glasgow, Glasgow, 1994), pp. 36–47.

11 Wendy Alexander, *First Ladies of Medicine: The Origins, Education and Destination of Early Women Graduates of Glasgow University* (Glasgow, 1987), pp. 41–42.
12 Kenneth Collins, *Go and Learn: The International Story of the Jews and Medicine in Scotland* (Aberdeen University Press, Aberdeen, 1987), p. 87. See Lists of Residents at the Western and Royal Infirmaries 1900–1945, Glasgow Health Board Archives.
13 Elizabeth Blackwell, *The Influence of Women in the Practice of Medicine* (Baltimore, 1890), p. 27. This publication is the text of her address in 1889 at the opening of the winter session of the London School of Medicine for Women. https://archive.org/details/39002086311165.med.yale.edu/page/28/mode/2up (accessed 1 April 2020).
14 Anne Digby, *The Evolution of British General Practice*, p. 173.
15 Ibid., pp. 175, 184. She quotes S. Taylor, *Good General Practice* (Nuffield Hospitals Trust, Oxford, 1954), pp. 52–54 on minor surgery: 'They do it extremely efficiently, with the neatness, aplomb and expertise which might otherwise go into dressmaking and embroidery'.
16 Eileen Janes Yeo, Medicine, Science and the Body in Lynn Abrams, Eleanor Gordon, Deborah Simonton, and Eileen Janes Yeo, *Gender in Scottish History Since 1700* (Edinburgh University Press, Edinburgh, 2006), pp. 140–169. Morrice McRae's book, *The National Health Service in Scotland: Origins and Ideals, 1900–1950* (Tuckwell Press, East Linton, East Lothian, 2003), makes no mention of women in medicine in Scotland during these five decades.
17 B. McKinstry, I. Colthart, K. Elliott, et al., The Feminization of the Medical Work Force, Implications for Scottish Primary Care: A Survey of Scottish General Practitioners, *BMC Health Services Research*, 6, 2006, p. 56.
18 Brian McKinstry, Are There Too Many Female Medical Graduates? Yes, *BMJ*, 336, 2008, p. 748.
19 Vanessa Heggie, Women Doctors and Lady Nurses, pp. 267–292.
20 E. Moberley Bell, *Storming the Citadel*, pp. 189–190.
21 Helen M. Dingwall, *A History of Scottish Medicine: Themes and Influence* (Edinburgh University Press, Edinburgh, 2003), p. 201.
22 Ibid., p. 202.
23 Morag C. Timbury and Maria A. Ratzer, Glasgow Medical Women 1951–4: Their Contribution and Attitude to Medical Work, *British Medical Journal*, 2 (5653), 1969, pp. 372–374.
24 Writing on behalf of the London Association of the Medical Women's Federation, F Lefford noted that equality of access to medical courses had not led to equality of access of employment. See F. Lefford, Prejudice against Women Doctors, *British Medical Journal (Clinical Research Edition)*, 294 (6575), 1987, p. 838.
25 Anne Digby, *The Evolution of British General Practice 1850–1948* (Oxford University Press, Oxford, 1999), p. 89.
26 Adrian Furnham and K. V. Petrides, Joanna Temple, Patient Preferences for Medical Doctor, *British Journal of Health Psychology*, 11, 2006, pp. 439–449.
27 E. J. Hopkins, Anne M. Pye, L. M. M. Solomon, and Sylvia Solomon, The Study of 'Patients' Choice of Doctor in an Urban Practice, *Journal of the Royal College of General Practitioners*, 14, 1967, p. 282.
28 Sally Nichols, Women's Preferences for Sex of Doctor: A Postal Survey, *Journal of the Royal College of General Practitioners*, 37 (305), 1987, pp. 540–543.

29 J. Graffy, Patient Choice in a Practice with Men and Women General Practitioners, *British Journal of General Practice*, 40, 1990, pp. 13–15; C. J. Heaton and J. T. Marquez, Patient Preferences for Physician Gender in the Male Genital/Rectal Exam, *Family Practice Research Journal*, 10 (2), 1990, pp. 105–115; Jan J. Kerssens, Jozien M. Bensing, and Margriet G. Abdela, Patient Preference for Genders of Health Professionals, *Social Science and Medicine*, 44, 1997, pp. 1531–1540.

30 A. V. D. Brink-Muinen, D. H. D. Bakker, and J. M. Bensing, Consultations for Women's Health Problems: Factors Influencing Women's Choice of Sex of General Practitioner, *British Journal of General Practitioners*, 44, 1994, pp. 205–210.

31 K. L. Bertakis, L. J. Helms, E. J. Callahan, R. Azari, and J. A. Robbins, The Influence of Gender on Physician Practice Style, *Medical Care*, 33, 1995, pp. 407–416.

32 C. S. Weisman and M. A. Teitelbaum, Physician Gender and the Physician Patient Relationship: Recent Evidence and Relevant Questions, *Social Science and Medicine*, 20, 1985, pp. 1119–1127.

33 Kathy Waller, Women Doctors for Women Patients? *British Journal of Medical Psychology*, 61, 1998, pp. 125–135.

34 D. Phillips and F. Brooks, Women Patients' Preferences for Female or Male GPs, *Family Practice*, 15, 1998, pp. 543–547.

35 Beth A. Plunkett, Priya Kohli, B. A. Magdy, and P. Milad, The Importance of Physician Gender in the Selection of an Obstetrician or a Gynecologist, *American Journal of Obstetrics and Gynecology*, 186 (5), 2002, pp. 926–928.

36 W. I. U. Ahmad, E. E. M. Kernohan, and M. R. Baker, Patients' Choice of General Practitioner: Influence of Patients' Fluency in English and the Ethnicity and Sex of the Doctor, *British Journal of General Practice*, 39, 1989, pp. 153–155.

37 Julian Tudor Hart, The Inverse Care Law, *Lancet*, 297 (7696), 1971, pp. 405–412. In 2006, Tudor Hart was awarded the inaugural Discovery Prize by the RCGP as 'a general practitioner who has captured the imagination of generations of GPs with his groundbreaking research'.

38 Olive Checkland and Margaret Lamb, editors, *Health Care as Social History: The Glasgow Case* (Aberdeen University Press, Aberdeen, 1982), p. 6. See also R. Elder, M. Kirkpatrick, W. Ramsay, et al., *The Scottish Government Long-term Monitoring of Health Inequalities* (The Scottish Government, Edinburgh, 2010); Measuring quality in primary medical services using data from SPICE. NHS National Services Scotland, Edinburgh, Scotland; 2007; NHS National Services Scotland, Information Services Division Measuring long-term conditions in Scotland, June 2008. www.isdscotland.org/isd/5658.html.

39 Quoted in *The Old Closes and Wynds of Glasgow*, 1900, www.bl.uk/collection-items/the-old-closes-and-streets-of-glasgow (accessed 1 May 2022).

40 D. Walsh, N. Bendel, R. Jones, and P. Hanlon, It's Not 'Just Deprivation': Why Do Equally Deprived UK Cities Experience Different Health Outcomes? *Public Health*, 124 (9), 2010, pp. 487–495.

41 D. Walsh, G. McCartney, C. Collins, M. Taulbut, and G. D. Batty, History, Politics and Vulnerability: Explaining Excess Mortality in Scotland and Glasgow, *Public Health*, 151, 2017, pp. 1–12.

42 Vera Carstairs and Russell Morris, *Deprivation and Health in Scotland* (Aberdeen University Press, Aberdeen, 1991).

43 Ibid., p. 214.

44 Ibid., p. 293. Just three miles away Pollokshields, G41, was category 1.
45 Vera Carstairs and Russell Morris, *Deprivation and Health in Scotland* (Aberdeen University Press, Aberdeen, 1991), pp. 152–154.
46 Graham Watt, *General Practitioners at the Deep End: The Experience and Views of General Practitioners Working in the Most Severely Deprived Areas of Scotland* (Royal College of General Practitioners, Occasional Paper 89). Most of the GPs on the steering group were based in Glasgow, two at the Govan Health Centre.
47 https://canmore.org.uk/site/44226/glasgow-1345-govan-road-southern-general-hospital (accessed 23 January 2019).
48 David Hamilton, *The Healers: A History of Medicine in Scotland* (Canongate, Edinburgh, 1981), pp. 229–233.
49 Ibid.
50 Providing capital for general practice: the GPFC, Briefing, *British Medical Journal*, 1999, pp. 1294–1295.
51 Marshall Marinker, Why Make People Patients? *Journal of Medical Ethics*, 1, 1975, pp. 81–84.
52 Marshall Marinker, 'What Is Wrong' and 'How We Know It': Changing Concepts of Illness in General Practice, in Irvine Loudon, John Horder, and Charles Webster, editors, *General Practice under the National Health Service 1948–1967* (Clarendon Press, London, 1998), pp. 65–91.
53 Michael Balint (1896–1970) was a Hungarian psychoanalyst who moved from Budapest to England in 1938. From 1950, Michael and Enid Balint developed Balint groups—where doctors discussed issues arising in general practice, focussing on the responses of the doctors to their patients. His books included *The Doctor, His Patient and the Illness* (Churchill Livingstone, London, 1957). Enid Balint and J. S. Norell, editors, *Six Minutes for the Patient: Interactions in General Practice Consultations* (RKP, London, 1973).
54 M. Balint, J. Hunt, D. Joyce, M. Marinker, and J. Woodard, *Treatment or Diagnosis: A Study of Repeat Prescriptions in General Practice* (Tavistock Press, London, 1970).
55 Marshall Marinker, Personal Paper: Writing Prescriptions Is Easy, *British Medical Journal*, 314, 1997, p. 747. Franz Kafka, *A Country Doctor*, trans. Siegfried Mortkovits, *Vitalis, Prague, 1970, p. 16. (Originally published in 1920 as Ein Landarzt.) That the issue of compliance transcends illness definitions and nationality see:* R. B. Haynes, W. D. Taylor, D. L. Sackett, and J. C. Snow, The Magnitude of Compliance and Non-Compliance, in R. B. Haynes, W. D. Taylor, and D. L. Sackett, editors, *Compliance in Health Care* (Johns Hopkins University Press, Baltimore, 1979), pp. 11–22; Royal Pharmaceutical Society of Great Britain, *From Compliance to Concordance: Toward Shared Goals in Medicine Taking* (RPS, London, 1997); R. B. Haynes, D. L. Sackett, E. S. Gibson, D. W. Taylor, B. C. Hackett, and R. S. Roberts, Improvement of Medication Compliance in Uncontrolled Hypertension, *Lancet*, 307 (7972), 1976, pp. 1265–1268; M. Rovelli, D. Palmeri, E. Vossler, S. Bartus, D. Hull, and R. Schweizer, Non-compliance in Organ Transplant Recipients, *Transplantation Proceedings*, 21, 1989, pp. 833–834.
56 M. Marinker, The Chameleon, the Judas Goat, and the Cuckoo (Yorkshire Oration, 1977), *Journal of the Royal College of General Practitioners*, 28, 1978, pp. 199–206.
57 Marshall Marinker, 'What Is Wrong' and 'How We Know It': Changing Concepts of Illness in General Practice, in Irvine Loudon, John Horder, and

Charles Webster, editors, *General Practice under the National Health Service 1948–1967* (London, 1998), p. 91.

58 I. R. MacWhinney, General Practice as an Academic Discipline: Reflections after a Visit to the United States, *Lancet*, 287 (7434), 1966, pp. 419–423.

59 Iona Heath, How Medicine Has Exploited Rationality at the Expense of Humanity, *British Medical Journal*, 355, 2016, i5705. https://doi.org/10.1136/bmj.i5705.

60 Bruce G. Link and Jo C. Phelan, Conceptualizing Stigma, *Annual Review of Sociology*, 27, 2001, pp. 363–385.

61 Cathy Campbell and Harriet Deacon, Unravelling the Contexts of Stigma: From Internalisation to Resistance to Change, *Journal of Community and Applied Social Psychology*, 16 (6), 2006, pp. 411–417.

62 A centenary reunion of the families of the Serbian boys was organised by George Heriot's School and held at the National Library of Scotland on 6th June 2016. The information on Dr George was obtained from the speech given there by his youngest daughter, Zora Buchanan, now living in Vancouver, Canada (JK).

63 It is possible that Stevan George may have made his way to the island of Corfu where he was picked up by a British boat.

64 Anne Digby, *The Evolution of British General Practice 1850–1948* (Oxford University Press, Oxford, 1999), pp. 130–133.

65 Ibid., pp. 132–133.

66 Laura Oren, The Welfare of Women in Laboring Families: England, 1860–1950, *Feminist Studies*, 1 (3/4), 1973, p. 116.

67 Anne Hardy, *Health and Medicine in Britain since 1860* (Palgrave, Basingstoke, 2001), p. 81.

68 Nick Bosanquet and Chris Salisbury, The Practice, in Irvine Loudon, John Horder, and Charles Webster, editors, *General Practice under the National Health Service 1948–1967* (Clarendon Press, London, 1998), pp. 46–50.

69 Anne Digby notes in *The Evolution of British General Practice*, p. 139, that a house and a surgery on a 'capital corner plot' was advantageous in attracting patients and was seen a prime asset in selling a practice.

70 A personal recollection is that sometimes a single word sufficed to explain a consultation. An example is of a consultation represented by a single word—a prescribable anti-spasmodic. This indicated a negative abdominal examination, following the history taking and the diagnosis of possible irritable bowel syndrome.

71 Forby (Scots): besides, in addition to.

72 Many friendly societies were set up during the nineteenth century to provide working people with health insurance and death benefits in return for small weekly payments. The Ancient Order of Rechabites is a friendly society which grew out of the temperance movement which promoted abstinence from alcohol.

3

Study Methodology

This oral history study, and its analysis, also aims to add to the growing body of material on the history of general medical practice in Britain.[1] It elicits the health care account of patients in one urban practice and allows for the reconstruction of history in the telling of the story of how patients understand health, its management and illness impacts on them and their family. Through the interviews, and their analysis, it plans to follow such issues as the doctor–patient relationship and the full range of clinical encounters that a general practitioner will follow in their lifetime.

The challenge of this study has been not just to analyse the testimonies. Paul Thompson lays emphasis on the personality of the interviewer who is collecting the oral history: the ability to listen and their respect for the participants.[2] Besides the oral recordings, Dr Ockrim's retirement 'Letters to No-one', only found after her death almost twenty years later, allow us to understand the importance of the study to her and how she interacted with her patients. In encountering these interviews, we can see the beauty of the recollections and the relationship between patients and doctors built up over many decades. As a former principal in the practice from 1977 until 2007, I knew almost all these former patients well and have for a long time wanted to give voice to these records of health care. Both Dr Ockrim and those she interviewed expected that their testimonies would be published in a narrative form at some stage. This encouraged participants to express clearly what they felt was important in their past encounters with the medical profession and to give an accurate account of the social context where they lived—even to situations which had caused them considerable distress. This oral history study illustrates the story of a doctor and her medical partnership while giving meaning to attitudes to gender, ethnic minorities and the social history of Glasgow's Ibrox and Govan.

People often can relate accurately distant memories, whereas lesser important and much more recent happenings are forgotten. The study includes some recollections where two people recall the same event and details do not always match. Some do corroborate each other, while we will have occasion to note how some memories have changed with time. Many studies have been done on age-related memory loss, a feature of normal ageing and different from the severe memory deficits found in Alzheimer's disease.[3]

Lise Abrams and Meagan Farrell review many studies related to language processing in the elderly.[4] They show that some researchers argue that the capacity of

DOI: 10.1201/9781003369301-3

working memory decreases as we age, and so we hold less information. Others show that older adults are better storytellers than younger adults. This may be, they suggest, because older adults have had more experience with telling stories throughout their life or just possess different goals for communicating, particularly in autobiographical situations. However, by focussing on an autobiography, they may come to give themselves a more central role than the original story might have indicated.

The data produced by the study, the collection of oral history interviews, forms a complex account of memories, beliefs, experiences and opinions. Such outputs are often described as qualitative data, as opposed to quantitative data where research focusses on analysing measurable numbers to produce conclusions. As Ritchie and Spencer note, the last two decades have seen a notable growth in the use of qualitative methods for applied social policy research.[5] Qualitative research seeks to understand the views and perspectives of the people being studied, and through careful analysis, it can provide a detailed understanding of complex social interactions which can have greater meaning than the numbers-oriented qualitative approaches.[6]

Qualitative data can be 'flexible' and 'exploratory'.[7] It can produce texts which foster the development and communication of ideas, generating conclusions in previously unexplored fields. Studies have considered the question of researcher bias as the qualitative researcher becomes part of the research process because they are interacting within the study.[8] This highlights the importance that the qualitative researcher be well educated and experienced in the research methodology. The background and personality of the researcher is also important. We reflected on the risks of observer bias as we planned the study, attended Paul Thompson's course and followed his guidelines.

Though the oral history interviews were conducted between 1989 and 1992, their serious analysis only began in 2009, two years after Dr Ockrim's death. When I began listening again to the interviews and rereading the transcripts, it became clear that many of the insights of twenty years earlier were of considerable importance, as was the way in which family memories stretched back to even earlier decades. The question of secondary analysis in qualitative research has been addressed by social scientists in many countries. Medjedović found that, though there have been concerns with this research strategy, the experience of expert researchers suggests that the problems associated with secondary analysis, such as ethical issues, do not necessarily constitute unsolvable obstacles.[9] Other researchers show that secondary analysis has potentially important implications for qualitative researchers who seek to investigate sensitive topics within health.[10]

Bornat addressed some of the questions generated or processes involved in the secondary analysis of archived oral history in a paper at the University of Essex in 2008.[11] These questions concern the effect of the passing of time, changed contexts for analysis and interpretation, and new ethical considerations. This study, with its analysis taking place three decades after the interviews, shows the benefits of this secondary approach. Louise Corti explains that the historian is used to the study of unfamiliar material that is unfamiliar to them.[12] She points out that re-using archived qualitative data enables further exploration of the data from a new perspective and allows comparative research to be carried out, for example, over time.[13]

In using the medium of oral history, relying on methods of recording and interpretation which have developed in recent years, this oral history project has enabled the study of many aspects of life and experience not found in the standard history books. In this study, we feature an example of the doctor and patients combining to lay out a display of health and social history. Studies have examined the effect of the testimonies on the interviewer, producing a view that there can be no objective history as there are always biases that are brought to the encounter.[14] This, says Valerie Yow, may extend to the interviewer focussing on the issues that they feel are the most important, but where, as in this case, the interviewer has had a personal relationship with those being interviewed over many years, or even decades, this can have a significantly positive effect.

Lynn Abrams, Professor of Modern History at the University of Glasgow, has observed that more than just collecting testimonies, oral history is about elucidating, interpreting and understanding the interaction between interviewer and interviewee.[15] She points out that while conducting an interview is a practical means of obtaining information about the past, in the process of eliciting and analysing the material, one is confronted by the oral history interview as an event of communication which demands that we find ways of comprehending not just *what* is said but also *how* it is said, *why* it is said and *what* it means. Oral history requires that one thinks about its theory.[16]

The content of oral history depends to a large extent on the way the interviewer asks the questions and how any previous relationship affects the answers. In this study, we were encouraged to see how the encounter with the doctor is recalled, sometimes many years later, confirming the importance of the patient's narrative.[17] For the most part, the voice of the interviewer has been omitted except in situations where the responses would have seemed stilted without it. In many cases, the responses reflect that the voice of the interviewee is replying to a question. Oral history represents a dialogue, and while the voices of the interviewees is the primary focus of the study, we cannot ignore the presence of the questioning, retired general practitioner, Dr Ockrim. However, her role in these interviews has been to guide the discussion without confronting patient memories. In a rare instance, her own opinions were carefully noted where she defended the ethos of the National Health Service where a participant suggested the superiority of private medicine in America. Everyone has their own way of looking at events and telling their story. Here, the voices of the interviewees are presented with as little interference as possible. Where interviewees record known facts imprecisely, this will be recorded in a footnote.

THE PROJECT OUTLINE

The project had four distinct phases which can be summarised as follows:

1. *Planning*: This began with the proposal for an oral history project with the retired general practitioner in conversation with former patients. The oral history testimonies were to be recorded and transcribed and a publication was to be generated. The Wellcome Trust agreed to fund the recording of the interviews and their transcriptions but with certain conditions attached, as described later. Literature reviews accompanied each stage of the project. Ethical approval was obtained from the Greater Glasgow Health Board Research Ethical Committee.

2. *Preparation*: This involved attendance at an oral history training seminar, creation of the questionnaires and selection of participants.
3. *Recording and Transcription*: Conducting the oral history, recording reviews, transcribing and evaluating transcript texts.
4. *Editing and Analysing*: During the recruitment and recording process, both the interviewer and I continuously reviewed the progress of the study, the recordings and the feedback from participants. More recently has come the analysis of material, the organising of texts in a thematic form and the creation of the book's structure and its text.

Conducting the Interviews

There was some early concern from the Wellcome Trust about the value of interviews carried out by the patients' former doctor, worried that the doctor–patient relationship might affect the way memories were conveyed. The Wellcome Trust paid for the purchase of high-quality Marantz recording equipment; an Amstrad PCW8512 word processor, then a new but very significant improvement on the standard typewriter; and the secretarial help to transcribe all the interviews. In addition, the grant was conditional on Dr Ockrim and me attending an oral medical history course organised by Professor Paul Thompson, at the University of Essex.[18] Paul Thompson (b. 1935) is a British sociologist and oral historian who held the position of Research Professor of Sociology at the University of Essex. He is regarded as a pioneer in social science research, particularly due to the development of life stories and oral history within sociology and social history. Professor Thompson's work has ensured that oral history has been increasingly recognised as a key factor in understanding the history of the recent past.[19] Course completion at the end of the week of study recognised Dr Ockrim as interviewer and me as project designer and eventual interpreter of the recordings.[20] The course emphasised the importance of allowing the voice of the participant to be heard and the interviewer to ask and direct the questions but otherwise to be a silent presence.

Selection of Patient and Staff Interviewees (1989)

The initial aim was to interview sixty patients chosen on the basis of the following:

1. range of medical, surgical and psychiatric conditions
2. experience of pregnancy and childbirth
3. representation of the ethnic and social mix of the practice (The practice population had around 12% of its patients from ethnic minority communities, particularly from Pakistan, and high levels of social deprivation, as measured by health indicators.)[21]

Letters were sent to just over one hundred patients in October 1989, reflecting the previously mentioned criteria. Because of the aim to give priority to the examination, the experience of women's health and especially maternity care provided in the practice, it was agreed that 60% of the letters would be sent to female patients and 40% to men. The letter gave an outline of the study proposal explaining that the interviews would be carried out by Dr Ockrim, who had recently retired as the senior partner in the practice.[22] These would be used by me to produce a history of the practice, creating an account of family medicine over the previous decades.

There was a very good response to the mailing, and it was decided to interview all those who had responded positively. Some seventy-nine oral histories were obtained between September 1989 and May 1992. When oral histories obtained from practice staff members are included, Dr Ockrim conducted about two or three histories a month. Given the relatively long lead time between invitation and interview, regular contact was kept with participants to ensure ongoing interest. The age range of the research participants was 31 years to 85 years (average 57.5 years), and most patients above the mean age had good recollections of conditions in practice before the establishment of the National Health Service and its operation during its first years. Fifty-five women (72%) and twenty-two men (28%) were interviewed, indicating a much higher acceptance of the invitation by women registered at the practice. In many ways, this study reflects the 1980s which saw the increasing development of the voice of women in oral history.[23] Two of the interviewees were born in Pakistan, and two more came from families that had immigrated to Scotland from Pakistan and India.

Conducting the Oral Histories

Patients could choose where the interviews would take place. Most took place in the surgery (Figure 3.1), which was perceived as a neutral place after Dr Ockrim had retired and no longer had a consulting room there. A few were conducted in the

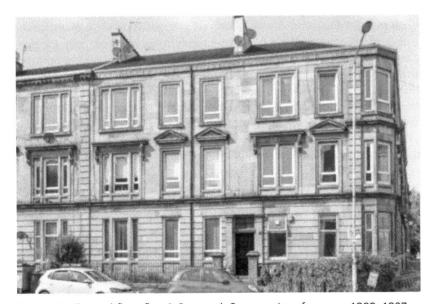

Figure 3.1 Ground-floor flat: 2 Cessnock Street—site of surgery 1929–1987.

patient's home, often reflecting a desire to extend hospitality in a way that would not have been appropriate before.

The interviews were planned around a semi-structured questionnaire which provided a basic framework with the questions directed by the interviewer.[24] There is an extensive literature on the use of semi-structured questionnaires, especially when dealing with health and illness. [25]

However, the flexible nature of the questionnaire allowed the patients considerable latitude in the topics covered. The aim of the questionnaire was to produce a free-flowing conversation between doctor and participants, and I have used the terms 'oral histories', 'interviews' and 'conversations' interchangeably.

The procedure followed the interview guide outlined by Paul Thompson.[26] The interviews usually lasted for up to two and a half hours, but a few lasted longer, as important recollections could take longer. No interview was curtailed through lack of time.

The questionnaire had four main sections:

a. *Opening Discussion*: these included the first memories of the practice, how it worked, the premises, personalities and events; pre- and post-NHS, hospital referrals, relative status of GPs and hospital doctors.
b. *Personal Health Issues*: main medical problems, attitudes to illness and how it was handled, impact of the illness on the patient and family, lesson learned.
c. *Family Health Issues*: illness in the family, how it was dealt with; support from medical and other agencies; experiences, lessons and impact.
d. *Health Care Changes*: attitudes to developments in modern medicine, GP teamwork and greater clinical responsibility by GPs for monitoring patient health.

Commonly, these topics reflected memories held for decades which were brought to mind during the course of following the structure of the questionnaire. The discussions, as shown later, begin with recollections of the practice, the premises and its workings, before dealing with personal, and then family, health issues. This allowed a gentle transition to the key individual memories. To conclude, participants were able to comment on changes in the delivery in medicine they had noticed over the years. Sometimes these also brought other personal questions into focus. Attitudes to access to the doctor were frequently expressed, and the growing importance of the concept of autonomy and a reduction in physician paternalism could be discussed with less of the emotion that the clinical topics sometimes engendered.

Though the interviews were not intended to have a therapeutic component, I will show that there is much to learn from the oral histories in the way in which clinical interviews are constructed. Though surgery consultations may be constrained by time, there are options for extended patient time, and many of the interviews point to the need for closure. Dr Ockrim was used to asking questions about health in all its aspects in a clinical context. For some of the participants, troubling memories of the past may have been allowed to have a sense of closure during the outlining of these events. Many studies have pointed to the potential for therapeutic outcomes in oral history through its revisiting of troublesome past events.[27]

As the interviews proceeded, we realised that much of the patients' memories were centred around the provision of care and how it had changed over the four decades since the founding of the National Health Service. Accordingly, Dr Ockrim and I decided to supplement the patient histories with those of the practice manager, reception staff and practice and district nurses. The dynamics of the interviews also marked a major difference from a medical consultation. Dr Ockrim would have seen each of her patients about the local average of four to five encounters a year, but additional contacts could have occurred with the consultations with their children, partners or elderly parents. Consultations in the open-access era averaged around six minutes, while the oral history interviews averaged around two and a half hours, longer than the Oral History Association guidelines which suggest between one and two hours.[28] No history was curtailed through time pressure.

There was time to understand not just the issue of the day but to have a full sense of everything that the participant represented, beliefs, opinions, illness and extended family connections, stories and legends. We will see how her approach, as illuminated in these interviews, shows how she viewed each research participant as unique individuals while never losing the focus on the clinical elements.

Oral History Study Records

Dr Ockrim kept records of her conversations in two forms. The limited space for notes on the semi-structured questionnaire attracted few comments. It was originally anticipated that the interviewer's notes would be kept on the questionnaire forms, but it became quickly apparent that this would be inadequate. Therefore, most of the feedback she recorded can be found on the cards in a small box file. This has ensured that we have detailed interviewer notes following the encounters and pointers to what seemed to be the most important elements. The card contains some details which can be a helpful introduction to the contents of the lengthy recordings and transcripts. They indicate aspects of how the session went and something of the interaction between the participants. This was of much value given the need for the interviewer and me to communicate effectively in the evaluation of the interview.

Paul Thompson describes the value of the careful evaluation of the interview once recorded and transcribed.[29] He also exhorts the interviewer to stay behind and chat after the session is completed, going forward 'with tact and caution'.[30] One note records that an interviewee requested that any mention of his anxiety recorded in a quoted text should be done with anonymity. In two cases, the interview ended with a request for Dr Ockrim to return for a further discussion. Another describes her arriving at the home of an interviewee to be met by the former patient's son. While waiting for his mother to appear, he confided that he was previously a drug addict but that his mother did not know. A few anonymised examples are given in the appendices.

Significant remarks on the card files sometimes include throwaway remarks after the recording had been completed. Thus, some family conflicts were mentioned only 'off the record'. One concerned a fostered child. Two referred to hospital experiences of relatives. In one case, there was a note about a relative who, it was alleged, had an accidental overdose of medication in hospital. In another post-interview remark, there was a belief expressed that a relative's death in hospital was euthanasia. One mentioned as he was leaving that his Alcoholics Anonymous group had once asked Dr David to come as a guest speaker and that he had done so.

The reflective time during the interviews allowed for an exchange of views on changes in practice and what patients look for in the encounter with their doctor. One patient (YT) missed the 'old days' when 'the doctor knew the whole family, he knew all about the family. He knew what the illnesses had been and what the granny had died of'.

The interviews with members of the practice and district nursing staff utilised a different questionnaire.[31] From the start, greater freedom was given to outline what they felt was important in their practice role and how their encounter with the patients played out. The questionnaire had the following seven sections, and the following elements were considered to be an aide-mémoire rather than a prescriptive list:

1. Memories of the old surgery in Cessnock Street and recollections of patients' attitudes to it. This might include the following:
   a. Working with a smaller staff and less paperwork (in the past)
   b. How the waiting room functioned in the open-access system
   c. The absence of a treatment room: the doctors doing all the tests, dressings, and so on
2. The nostalgia felt by many patients to the old surgery despite the clear lack of facilities available in the new building.
3. Incidents remembered.
4. How the staff have coped with patients who have severe social problems, especially drug addiction and alcoholism. Problems at the reception window.
5. The practice policy of open access, with morning appointments only beginning as the study began and full appointments (morning and evening) scheduled to start in February 1993, after the study was completed.
6. Impact on practice staff of new GP contracts and their views if they have improved the standards of care.
7. The practice functioned for many years with four doctors and one person in the office. How has the move from the cottage industry to the then present setup been managed?

THE DATA AND HOW IT WAS ORGANISED

The study generated around 200 hours of recordings, and the transcription took over 500 hours. This produced more than 2,000 pages of transcripts, comprising more than half a million words, laboriously printed out at the time on the Amstrad word processor. The Amstrad used an early computer programme called Locoscript, and this was converted to Microsoft Word format in 2008.

The organisation of the vast amount of material was a complex task. Clinical topics, for example, were scattered through all the interviews. Arranging these topics

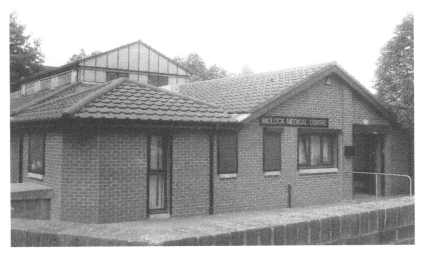

Figure 3.2 Midlock Medical Centre: opened February 1987.

into common themes and individual diseases along with personal viewpoints and memories was time-consuming. Within the common themes, such as practice arrangements, there were further subdivisions which required setting into common topics. This included attitudes to open-access and appointment systems, home visits and childbirth. The process was very tedious but had to be completed before organised study of the material could begin.

In 2014, with concern about the long-term survival of the audiotapes, the oral history recordings and the transcripts were deposited at the Scottish Oral History Centre (SOHC) which was established at the University of Strathclyde, Glasgow, in 1995. The recordings have been digitised but remain accessible only with the approval of the Midlock Medical Centre (Figure 3.2). SOHC seemed to be a good home as it has been involved in a wide range of teaching, research and outreach activities which they had designed primarily to encourage the use of best practice in oral history methodology in Scotland.[32]

Inclusion of Material

The choice of material from the transcripts, representing barely a tenth of the total word count, was also a complex task. Many of the testimonies said much the same things on a variety of topics. Sometimes a key sentence or paragraph could be embedded in a digression on an entirely different topic. Not all the material that was fascinating, from a social point of view, could be used. At the same time, I was mindful of Paul Thompson's words that oral history can give a central place to the people who made and experienced history, through their own words.[33]

The quotes from the transcripts cover the full range of the experience of general practice, its organisation and its medical practices. While the interviewer took great care to remain the silent facilitator, the interactions between former doctor and patient show great respect for each other and has much to say about the aspiration by one female practitioner who saw herself as part of the movement of women into Scottish professional life.

Abrams's comments on the 'what, how and why it is said' and 'what it means' are addressed in the study of the transcripts and accompany each of the testimony abstracts. In a few places, I have added some explanations and clarifications from insights made during my own experiences of over thirty years as a partner in the practice, for nearly half of which, from 1976 to 1989, was as a colleague of Dr Ockrim.

The categories of the interview were as follows:

a. **Historical**: this comprises the background of Dr Ockrim as a woman doctor at a time when there was much prejudice for females to face; the story of Dr Stevan George, the Serbian refugee who founded the practice; and the beginnings of the National Health Service. The material for this topic came exclusively from the oral histories of the former patients of Dr George and Dr Ockrim.

b. **Organisational**: practice arrangements, including its management, open access and appointments and house calls. Here, the material came from testimonies from staff members as well as former patients of the practice.

c. **Clinical**: the full range of material related to child health, obstetrics and gynaecology, medicine, surgery, psychiatry, infectious diseases and addictions. These clinical topics came from Dr Ockrim's patients as they recalled what was important in their health experiences.

d. **Stigma and Marginalisation**: stigma was found to be associated particularly with pre-NHS institutions, tuberculosis, mental health and addictive behaviours.

   Ethnic and religious minorities in the practice suffered from marginalisation within the wider society and from access to their specific health needs which did not always receive appropriate NHS funding.

The first step in organising the material was to identify accounts related to the four sections just mentioned. This involved careful study of each of the interviews, including all the questions and responses related to the topics. From there, the quotations were edited, retaining the essential meaning of the testimony in as concise a form as possible. Finally, the material was further refined, ensuring its flow. There was careful attention to retaining the language of the interviewees and less common dialect words have been explained. The texts also had to be used in a way which make it extremely difficult, if not impossible, to identify the interviewees' recording of sensitive material. Since the interviews were carried out, more than one-third have died and further one-fifth have moved away, but attempts have been made to contact patients still within the practice to show how their testimonies will be used.

All the staff members agreed to waive anonymity, as did two of the other participants. I have given careful thought to how the original names of interviewees should be used. Some researchers feel that it is appropriate to use the real names of those interviewed as it gives an additional degree of authenticity. Bornat describes the issues related to confidentiality, which matters more in a health care setting.[34] She notes that the British Copyright Act of 1988 gives copyright of the words to the participants and of the recordings to the responsible person or organisation conducting the study. SOHC advice was to anonymise the names, and the two options were using a code, with numbers and letters, or providing substitute names. My preference has been for using a code.

Producing a flowing narrative for this oral history is complicated by the way people speak—sometimes sentences are truncated, and stories are interrupted when the telling leads the narrator on to something else which has just been recalled and is also of importance. Bartlett has said that 'in a world of constantly changing environment, literal recall is extra-ordinarily unimportant. . . . Every time we make it, it has its own characteristics.'[35]

Interpreting the Material

Researchers have come to accept that there is more to testimonies than established fact. Ruth Finnegan counsel us to remember that oral history is not 'a collection of empirical data transmitted by some mechanical process.'[36] Accepting minor inaccuracies does not detract from how the past was understood.[37] There were subtle differences in recalling of the same events by different observers, such as the heroism of Dr George during the Clydeside Blitz, the question of an award for his wartime work and his subsequent departure for the Bahamas. Dr George was the founder of the practice, and his story is recalled by study participants in a later chapter. We will see how individual memories function in corroborating the main events while we note some minor details of difference which add nuance to the story.

In some instances, the memories of patients interviewed in this study were challenged. There were two occasions where a central character in the recollection, namely the practice manager, was said to have made the diagnosis personally. The practice manager vigorously denied, both at the time and in a later evaluation session, that she would ever have given a patient the results of a test or suggested a diagnosis. We might conclude that the stories might indicate how the practice manager was seen to have been a significant and authoritative person in the practice.

Sometimes memories might stray into gossiping, usually described as discussion of a third party who is not present. This was a behaviour that one participant, who had been a patient of the practice as well as a local pharmacist, would not be drawn into, whether the information was positive or negative. She described the care she had taken to avoid getting involved in a conversation about the merits of some local doctors and their prescribing. She recalled that 'You got one or two coming in complaining and then the next person would come in and talk about the same doctor, and say they were marvellous' (ISe). Such instances are frequent. Two of the small number of comments about the abilities of local hospital consultants concerned just one orthopaedist. He had been described by one patient as one of the most kind and caring doctors she had ever encountered, while another considered that he was the rudest person 'on the face of the earth'. We will see how two interviewees recalled the occasion around 1950, with some differing details, when Dr Ockrim had no patients waiting for her while the waiting room was full of patients waiting for Dr Collins.

Producing an understanding of the material involved a review of the various aspects of how handling oral history is dealt with. This involves the following.

UNDERSTANDING THE DOCTOR–PATIENT RELATIONSHIP

This book follows the relationship between one general practitioner and a representative sample of her former patients. While the study gave Dr Ockrim the possibility to follow the story of the participants in an extended session, the doctor–patient relationship derives from the shorter and outcome-focussed surgery consultation. The study of this relationship has received much attention, and it would be impossible to understand the dynamic between doctor and participant in these interviews without reference to the work of Michael Balint (1896–1970). Balint was the pioneer of understanding the patient's story in the context of, as the title of his seminal book described it, *The Doctor, His Patient and the Illness*, (Churchill Livingstone, London, 1957).[38] Balint had emphasised the importance of the doctors need to 'learn to listen', getting the physician to view and experience empathically the patient's world and their situation within it.[39] Balint believed that the result of persistent hard work on both sides to gain the other's confidence formed part of an important domain for research 'which medical science has neglected'. He noted that little or no attention had been given to the patient's subjective experience of improvement or sense of resolution of their illness and the doctor's sense of satisfaction with having effectively understood and addressed the patient's illness describing 'every illness is also the "vehicle" of a plea for love and attention'.[40]

Marshall Marinker (1930–2019), Professor of General Practice at the University of Leicester, was a participant in Michael Balint's groups, and his work on the analysis of the doctor–patient relationship set the agenda for generations of general practitioners. He pointed out that science alone could not encompass the whole story as he considered this:

> the view of man (or woman) as an object and the belief that the clinical task is to distinguish the clear message of the disease from the interfering noise of the patient as a person—constitutes a threat to medical humanism.[41]

Meyerscough describes the short clinical interviews as requiring a balance between involvement and detachment, with doctors tending to tip the balance towards detachment.[42] He suggests that involvement can seem burdensome and threatening and that its risks of greater intensity could lead to burnout. Interviews also give a lively sense of ease and comfort where difficult issues, including often considered taboo subjects as death and sexuality, can be considered in an atmosphere of mutual respect.

The dynamic of the clinical encounter between doctor and patient was further explored by Elliot Mishler (1924–2018) who was a professor of social psychology at the Harvard Medical School. Mishler had a significant influence on the development of narrative psychology, the study of how human beings construct stories to deal with experiences. Consequently, I believe that it is important to understand his insights and the light they cast on the encounter between physician and patient. His article titled 'Patient stories, narratives of resistance and the ethics of humane care: a la recherche du temps perdu', published in 2005, examines in detail the doctor–patient relationship and what that relationship can teach us about the various elements that make up a successful consultation.[43] This paper followed another article, published the previous year, which had analysed the contrast between two lines of inquiry in the health care field and their respective ethical priorities: the study of the patient–physician relationship, guided by an ethic of humane care and research on the health impact of social and economic inequality framed within an ethic of social justice.[44]

Mishler felt that there was a lack of attention by health care practitioners and researchers concerned primarily with patient–practitioner communication and how the relationship impacted on indices of morbidity and mortality, and access to care. He called this the 'unjust world problem' to characterise the disconnect between 'humane care' and 'social justice'. This American version of the 'inverse care law' would be of benefit if doctors, and other health care practitioners, could bring humane care and social justice into their medical practice.

Mishler's focus was on the quality of the interpersonal relationship between physicians and their patients, often based on issues of power and hierarchy, and its possible impact of this relationship to health care inequalities.[45] He noted that major changes had occurred from the 1980s with 'a phenomenal growth of interest in patients' stories in the health care field'. This followed societal unease with a 'highly technological form of clinical practice' which led to a downgrading of the time that doctors spent in talking to or listening to their patients.[46]

One of Mishler's findings was that there was very little reference in studies of patients' stories in clinical encounters to their daily experiences of living under conditions of poverty, oppression or social exclusion.[47] This could be, he felt, the result of collusion between doctor and patient and declared that 'We need exemplars accounts of efforts that not only include patients' stories in transcripts of clinical encounters . . . but that engage them critically as socially positioned persons with alternative understandings of what has been happening to them'.[48] This is what this book aims to address.

UNDERSTANDING THE MEDICAL NARRATIVE

Following on from the doctor–patient relationship, this oral history study has a special contribution to make what is being called narrative medicine.[49] A story usually has a narrator and a listener, and the doctor–patient relationship can form one example of the narrative. In the analysis of the participants' testimonies, we can see how these extended memories give a detailed exposition of their health life stories. Thus, the analysis of these memories leans also on what we learn from the newly emergent discipline of narrative medicine. We will understand what separates the oral history interview from the surgery or home-based consultation and reflect on what each can teach the other in the retelling of these stories.

Narrative medicine has become an important feature of general practice from the mid-1980s. There has increasingly been a focus on narrative in medicine, where the practitioner understands the health concerns of their patient and creates a connection between the two. This focus was in its early stage when the oral history project began. This aspect of the interaction between doctor and patient has received increased attention, relating to many themes such as ethical issues and relationship studies and drawing inspiration from literary studies and the humanities.[50] As medicine becomes more scientific, the stories that doctors and patients tell still show a contemporary relevance. Narrative medicine was understood to be the pathway towards rational treatment, based upon understanding and knowledge of hidden causes of ill health. The interviews also follow a narrative trend but with the aim of understanding a collective voice for the patient experience, telling a story for the wider public which would not otherwise be told. The general practitioner is in a privileged position being able to follow the medical and social course of a patient's life for many decades. This has benefits both in narrative medicine and oral medical history.

In the introduction to their book *Narrative Based Medicine: Dialogue and Discourse in Clinical Practice*, Trisha Greenhalgh and Brian Hurwitz indicate that, in the diagnostic encounter, narratives are not just where patients experience illness, but they set a patient-centred agenda.[51] Greenhalgh and Hurwitz considered that the search for meaning, which was at the heart of narrative in medicine, could be challenging for doctors, based as it is in literature rather than science.[52] Consequently, they say, 'doctors and patients often assign very different meanings to the same sequence of events'. However, Heath notes that narrative occupies a special place in general practice as it is the long-term relationship between doctor and patient which underpins primary care.[53] She also considers that narrative takes time and requires the listener to acknowledge the longitudinal nature of the patient's experiences. Hurwitz has pointed out that the traditional medical view of the consultation is to see it as an opportunity to fashion a clinical case history. This then becomes progressively abstracted from the patient's control, and the context of its original telling may end in case conferences and the medical literature.[54]

The strength of this study is to see the patient maintained at the centre of the story, while the narrative is expressed in a medical context of health care facilities and clinical outcomes. As the general practitioner also has intimate knowledge of the patient's circumstances, their medical history and family background, it could be argued that narrative has long been the basis of doctor–patient relationship. In this study with interviews lasting for around two hours, all the aspects of their medical history are enriched by their attitudes to the doctor and the illness. Launer, one of the leading figures in describing the medical narrative in Britain, points out that while doctors may believe in their explanation of symptoms of diagnosis as unshakable truths, they can prove to be as transient or evolutionary as the stories the patients bring to their doctors about their own lives. In this study, we encounter many different views of the patient understanding of 'medical diagnosis'.

While doctor's stories involve the interpretation of the illness to the patient, setting the context for diagnosis and treatment, Launer has noted that doctors may still unwittingly ignore or disqualify people's realities by failing to catch many of the exact words, phrases and metaphors with which they weave their stories.[55] In this study, the family doctor builds on years or decades of shared experiences to allow for the flow of patient memories, expressed in their own idiom. Such studies can help our understanding, doctor and patient, of what we tell each other in the consulting room.

Charon also suggests that as the empathic physician listens to the patient, she or he follows the narrative thread of the story, imagines the situation of the teller (the biological, familial, cultural and existential situation), recognises the multiple and often contradictory meanings of the words used and the events described. With these skills, the patient can build up trust in the doctor and enable the therapeutic encounter to proceed.

Launer and Lindsey have noted that certain ideas that are deeply ingrained in general practice are now under serious attack, especially where doctors make unchallenged hypotheses about the patient's 'hidden agenda' to speculate about the psychosomatic nature of symptoms or to choose professional priorities over the patient's.[56] They say that while accepting that experts must give advice about matters that lie within the domain of professional knowledge, critics are also drawing attention to the abuse of power that can occur when experts operate in areas such as family, culture and gender. At the same time, Richard McKay has pointed this out:

> medicine and health care are deeply embedded social enterprises and many aspects of human health are shaped by a wide range of non-medical factors. We use medicine and healing as lenses for exploring different experiences of health and disease, which are affected by class, race, ethnicity, gender and sexuality.[57]

VALIDITY OF THE DATA

Oral history allows for more than just the recovery of undocumented historical events. The narrative, created from the hundreds of hours of recordings and the thousands of pages of transcript, has also given expression to otherwise unheard voices and their concerns. We hear the opinions of those who wanted their babies born at home and access to the surgery to be open on a first-come basis. We hear the anguish of lives blighted by alcohol and illicit substances, cancer and tuberculosis. Above all, we find the voices of those who place their trust in their family doctor. We hear those who recognised in their doctor someone who would argue for their rights, enable the disadvantaged to find their way and help the curious to follow their dreams. At the same time, we discover some discrepancies in various accounts, especially where more than one person recalls the same event.

Testimonies from oral histories are, by their nature, very subjective. Consequently, many researchers have noted that, just as in other types of evidence, the material recorded in oral history interviews will display varying levels of accuracy, requiring researchers to take care in examining their sources. Memories may even clash with the prior understandings of the researcher. Paul Thompson points to the paradox at the heart of oral history, saying that 'any historical work suffers the inevitable disadvantage of having to work from the real cases available rather than created from specially created experiments'.[58]

Thompson also considers that, in oral history, 'wrong' statements are still psychologically 'true' and that this truth may be equally as important as factually reliable accounts. Lawrence Langer also accepted that the value of recalled memories achieves a gravity that surpasses the concern with accuracy.[59] Mark Roseman noted in his oral history of Holocaust survivors that he encountered 'significant patterns of discrepancy' relating to minor inaccuracies in testimony, which could be related to the trauma of the event.[60]

Patients might not be able to recount the precise year that major events in their lives occurred, but as Alessandro Portelli notes, oral history adds much more than such details. It contributes, he says, by adding meaning: 'an active process of creation of meanings'.[61] He points out that what makes oral history different is the speaker's subjectivity[62] and its sometimes divergence from 'facts' through participants' imagination.[63] However, he points out that just as oral histories may describe distant events, historians often use written sources which were written long after the actual events.

In this chapter, we have considered the various issues involved in conducting an oral history study, examining how the testimonies have been used—analysed and interpreted—looking at the validity of the evidence, how participants were chosen, and their recollections recorded. Memories can be flawed, but recollections form part of identity, and the past has lessons for the present and future. This extensive collection of medical and social narratives can now be considered through the prism of practice organisation, stigma and marginalisation, and clinical issues.

NOTES

1 Irvine Loudon, John Horder, and Charles Webster, *General Practice under the National Health Service 1948–1977* (Clarendon Press, Oxford, 1998). The book provides an invaluable guide to general practice in the first years of the National Health Service, but the evidence provided comes from medical practitioners or social scientists rather than patients.
2 Paul Thompson, *Oral History: The Voice of the Past* (3rd edition) (Oxford University Press, Oxford, 1988), p. 116.
3 See, for example, A. E. Budson and B. H. Price, Memory Dysfunction, *New England Journal of Medicine*, 352 (7), 2005, pp. 692–699.
4 Lise Abrams and Meagan T. Farrell, Language Processing in Normal Aging, https://web.archive.org/web/20121224080934/www.psych.ufl.edu/~abrams/Research/abrams_farrell_11.pdf (accessed 17 March 2020).
5 Jane Ritchie and Liz Spencer, Qualitative Data Analysis for Applied Policy Research, in A. Michael Huberman, and Matthew B. Miller, editors, *The Quantitative Researcher's Companion* (Sage Publications, Thousand Oaks, 2002), pp. 305–306.
6 Joan E. Dodgson, *About Research*, pp. 355–358.
7 Melissa E. Graebner, Jeffrey A. Martin, and Philip T. Roundy, Qualitative Research: Cooking without a Recipe, *Strategic Organization*, 10 (3), 2002, pp. 276–284.
8 John W. Creswell and Cheryl N. Poth, *Qualitative Inquiry and Research Design: Choosing among Five Approaches* (SAGE Publications, Thousand Oaks, 2017).

9 I. Medjedović, Secondary Analysis of Qualitative Interview Data: Objections and Experiences. Results of a German Feasibility Study, *Forum Qualitative Sozialforschung/Forum: Qualitative Social Research*, 12 (3), 2011.

10 There is a considerable literature on this topic. Tim May, editor, Qualitative Interviewing: Asking, Listening and Interpreting, in *Qualitative Research in Action* (Sage Research Methods), https://methods.sagepub.com/base/download/BookChapter/qualitative-research-in-action/n10.xml (accessed 22 March 2022). See also A. Thomson, Four Paradigm Transformations in Oral History, *Oral History Review*, 34 (1), 2007, pp. 49–70; P. Leavy, *Oral History: Understanding Qualitative Research* (Oxford University Press, Oxford, 2011); V. J. Janesick, *Oral History for the qualitative Researcher: Choreographing the Story* (Guildford Press, New York, 2010); T. Long-Sutehall, M. Sque, and J. Addington-Hall, Secondary Analysis of Qualitative Data: A Valuable Method for Exploring Sensitive Issues with an Elusive Population? *Journal of Research in Nursing*, 16 (4), 2011, pp. 335–344. See also the exploration of ethical issues in Sally Thorne, Ethical and Representational Issues in Qualitative Secondary Analysis, *Qualitative Health Research*, 8 (4), 1998, pp. 547–555.

11 Joanna Bornat, Crossing Boundaries with Secondary Analysis: Implications for Archived Oral History Data, www.restore.ac.uk/archiving_qualitative_data/projects/archive_series/documents/ArchivedEthicsandArchivesEssex19-0-.08JBornat_000.pdf (accessed 20 March 2022).

12 Louise Corti, Qualitative Archiving and Data Sharing: Extending the Reach and Impact of Qualitative Data, 2006, http://repository.essex.ac.uk/24479/1/iqvol293corti.pdfCorti (accessed 20 March 2022).

13 L. Cort, Re-using Archived Qualitative Data—Where, How, Why? *Archival Science*, 7, 2007, pp. 37–54.

14 Valerie Yow, 'Do I Like Them Too Much?' Effects of the Oral History Interview on the Interviewer and Vice Versa, in Robert Perks and Alistair Thomson, editors, *The Oral History Reader* (2nd edition) (Routledge, Abingdon, 2006), pp. 54–72.

15 Lynn Abrams, *Oral History Theory* (2nd edition, eBook) (Routledge, London and New York, 2018), p. 21.

16 Ibid., p. 1.

17 Alessandro Portelli, What Makes Oral History Different, in Robert Perks and Alastair Thomson, *The Oral History Reader* (2nd edition, 2006) (Routledge, London, 1st edition, 1998), p. 39.

18 Additional lecturers were Ludmilla Jordanova, the author of many texts regarding the history of science, thinking, gender and art; and Elizabeth (Tilli) Tansey, Emerita Professor of the History of Medicine, best known for her role in the Wellcome Trust's witness seminars.

19 See, for example, Bill Williams, *Book Review: The Voice of the Past*, Oral History, 7 (1), 1979, pp. 63–65.

20 Paul Thompson is the founding editor of the journal *Oral History* and the founder of the National Life Story Collection at the British Library National Sound Archive, London. His publications include *Oral History: The Voice of the Past*, 1978; *Listening for a Change: Oral Testimony and Development* (Panos Publications, London, 1993); *The Edwardians: The Remaking of British Society* (Weidenfeld and Nicolson, London, 1975) and, most recently, with Ken Plummer and Neli Demireva, *Pioneering Social Research: Life Stories of a Generation* (Bristol University Press, Bristol, 2022). See also Paul Thompson,

Oral History and the History of Medicine: A Review, *Social History of Medicine*, 4 (2), 1991, pp. 371–383.

21 Vera Carstairs and Russell Morris, *Deprivation and Health in Scotland* (Aberdeen University Press, Aberdeen, 1991), pp. 4–11.

22 Letter in Appendix.

23 Susan Armitage and Sherna Berger Gluck, Reflections on 'Women's Oral History: An Exchange, *Frontiers: A Journal of Women Studies*, 19 (3), 1998, pp. 1–11.

24 See Appendix.

25 J. Corbin and J. M. Morse, The Unstructured Interactive Interview: Issues of Reciprocity and Risks When Dealing with Sensitive Topics, *Qualitative Inquiry*, 9 (3), 2003, pp. 335–354; Michal Mahat-Shamir, Robert A. Neimeyer, and Shani Pitcho-Prelorentzos, Designing In-depth Semi-structured Interviews for Revealing Meaning Reconstruction after Loss, *Death Studies*, 45, 2021, pp. 83–90. See also Jacqueline Low, Structured and Unstructured Interviews in Health Research, in Mike Saks and Judith Alsop, editors, *Researching Health: Qualitative, Quantitative and Mixed Methods* (Sage Publications, 2013). (Chapter 5).

26 Paul Thompson, *Oral History: The Voice of the Past* (3rd edition), Interview guidelines are on pp. 198–204, while a more detailed scheme for interviews is on pp. 296–306.

27 This is discussed in a number of different articles in the *Oral History Reader*: Daniel James, Listening in the Cold, p. 98; Interviewing Introduction, p. 118, Kathryn Anderson, Dana C. Jack, Learning to Listen, p. 135; Mark Klempner, Interviews with Trauma Survivors, pp. 198–210; Joanna Bornat, Reminiscence and Oral History, p. 459. See also R. Harris, S. Harris, Therapeutic Uses of Oral History Techniques in Medicine, *International Journal of Aging and Human Development*, 12 (1), 1981, pp. 27–34, who cite practical applications of oral history techniques in clinical medical practice especially in old age.

28 www.oralhistory.org/about/.

29 Paul Thompson, *Oral History: The Voice of the Past* (3rd edition), Chapter 9: the Making of History, pp. 234–265. Similar advice is given in Kathryn Anderson and Dana C. Jack, Learning to Listen: Interview Techniques and Analyses in *The Oral History Reader*, pp. 129–142.

30 Paul Thompson, *Oral History: The Voice of the Past* (3rd edition), pp. 211–212.

31 See Appendix.

32 Angela Bartie and Arthur McIvor, Oral History in Scotland, *The Scottish Historical Review*, 92 (234), 2013, Supplement: The State of Early Modern and Modern Scottish Histories, pp. 108–136.

33 Paul Thompson, *Oral History: The Voice of the Past* (3rd edition), p. 3.

34 Joanna Bornat, Reminiscence and Oral History, in *The Oral History Reader* (2nd edition), pp. 468–469.

35 F. C. Bartlett, *Remembering, A Study in Experimental and Social Psychology* (Cambridge University Press, Cambridge, 1932), p. 240, http://nwkpsych. rutgers.edu/~jose/courses/578_mem_learn/2012/readings/Bartlett_1932.pdf (accessed 17 March 2020).

36 Ruth Finnegan, Family Myths, Memories and Interviewing in Robert Perks, Alistair Thomson, editors, *The Oral History Reader*, 2nd edition, p.180.

37 Mark Roseman, Surviving Memory: Truth and Inaccuracy in Holocaust Testimony, in *The Oral History Reader*, pp. 230–243; also see the section on 'Should we believe oral history sources' in Alessandro Portelli's chapter 'What Makes Oral History Different', in *The Oral History Reader*, pp. 37–38.

38 Alan H. Johnson, Clive D. Brock, Ashleigh Zacarias, The Legacy of Michael Balint, *International Journal of Psychiatry in Medicine*, 47 (3), 2014, pp. 175–192.

39 Michael Balint, *The Doctor, His Patient and the Illness* (Churchill Livingstone, London, 1957), pp. 121, 250.

40 Ibid., p. 276.

41 Marshall Marinker, The Narrative of Hilda Thomson, in Trisha Greenhalgh and Brian Hurwitz, *Narrative Based Medicine: Dialogue and Discourse in Clinical Practice* (BMJ Books, London, 1998), pp. 103–109.

42 Philip R. Myerscough, *Talking to Patients: A Basic Clinical Skill* (Oxford Medical Publication, OUP, New York, 1989), p. 135.

43 Elliot G. Mishler, Patient Stories, Narratives of Resistance and the Ethics of Humane Care: A La Recherche Du Temps Perdu, *Health: An Interdisciplinary Journal for the Social Study of Health, Illness and Medicine*, 9 (4), 2005, pp. 431–451.

44 E. G. Mishler, The Unjust World Problem: Towards an Ethics of Advocacy for Health Care Providers and Researchers, *Communication, Medicine, and Ethics*, 1, 2004, pp. 97–104.

45 Elliot G. Mishler, Patient Stories, Narratives of Resistance and the Ethics of Humane Care, p. 432.

46 Ibid., p. 435.

47 Ibid., p. 439.

48 E. G. Mishler, Validation in Inquiry-Guided Research: The Role of Exemplars in Narrative Studies, *Harvard Educational Review*, 60, 1990, pp. 415–442.

49 See, for example, the following editorial: John Launer, Narrative-based Medicine: A Passing Fad or a Giant Leap for General Practice? *British Journal of General Practice*, 53 (487), 2003, pp. 91–92.

50 Anne Hudson Jones, Narrative in Medical Ethics, *British Medical Journal*, 318, 1999, p. 2.

51 Trisha Greenhalgh and Brian Hurwitz, *Narrative Based Medicine*, p. 7.

52 Ibid., pp. 10–12.

53 Iona Heath, Following the Story: Continuity of Care in General Practice, in Trisha Greenhalgh and Brian Hurwitz, editors, *Narrative Based Medicine*, pp. 83–92.

54 Brian Hurwitz, History and Narrative in Clinical Medicine, *Lancet*, 356 (9247), 2000, pp. 2086–2089.

55 John Launer, Narrative-based Medicine: A Passing Fad or a Giant Leap for General Practice? *British Journal of General Practice*, 2003, pp. 91–92. See also John Launer, Narrative and Mental Health in Primary Care, in Trisha Greenhalgh and Brian Hurwitz, editors, *Narrative Based Medicine: Dialogue and Discourse in Clinical Medicine* (BMJ Books, London, 1998).

56 John Launer and Caroline Lindsey, Training for Systemic General Practice: A New Approach from the Tavistock Clinic, *British Journal of General Practice*, 47, 1997, pp. 453–456.

57 Richard A. McKay, Why Do We Do What We Do?: The Values of the Social History of Medicine, *Social History of Medicine: The Journal of the Society of the Social History of Medicine*, 33 (1), 2020, p. 8.

58 Paul Thompson, *The Voice of the Past: Oral History* (2nd edition) (Oxford University Press, Oxford, 1988), p. 252.

59 Lawrence L. Langer, *Holocaust Testimonies: The Ruins of Memory* (Yale University, New Haven, 1991), p. xv.

60 Mark Roseman, Surviving Memory: Truth and Inaccuracy in Holocaust Testimony, in Robert Perks and Alistair Thomson, editors, *The Oral History Reader* (2nd edition) (Routledge, London and New York, 1998), pp. 230–243.
61 Alessandro Portelli, What Makes Oral History Different? in Robert Perks and Alistair Thomson, editors, *The Oral History Reader* (2nd edition) (Routledge, London and New York, 1998), pp. 32–42.
62 A. Portelli, On the Peculiarities of Oral History, *History Workshop Journal*, 12, 1981, p. 99.
63 Ibid., p. 100.

4

Practice Organisation

ISSUES IN PRACTICE ORGANISATION

Although the original plan for the oral history study was based exclusively on patient contacts, we soon agreed on the need to record further interviews with members of the practice team, that is the office staff, the first practice-based nurse and one of the attached district nurses. These interviews help to flesh out the organisational arrangements for the practice and describe their views of the context in which the patient contacts took place. They provide a window into conditions in general practice and the developing role of receptionists and practice manager. We can also see the first signs of the increasing trend of more knowledgeable patients who were becoming more likely to criticise their doctors.[1] This trend has only accelerated after the interviews were completed, as access to the internet and social media increased.

These organisational issues will be considered in three sections:

Access: This shows how patients accessed health care in the surgery and at home, and the extensive literature on patient access will form a background to practice arrangements for acute illness and for continuity of care in chronic illness.

Management: We consider how the practice operated, both in Cessnock Street and at the purpose-built Midlock Medical Centre, with its staff—at first just clerical and administrative—and later, with clinical support. It was the key role of the receptionists which delivered many of the changes that came to be accepted as good practice. These included forming the interface with patients and providing access to the doctors, organising the office paperwork which ensured NHS funding and facilitating the work practices of the doctors.

Working Practices: At the time of the study, there were around 9,000 patients in the practice or 2,250 patients per doctor which was higher than the Scottish average. Gradually, the recruitment of additional doctors on part-time contracts and the increased demands of new NHS contracts led to this number dropping close to national averages. At the same time, the number of supportive office and clinical staff increased.

DOI: 10.1201/9781003369301-4

THE CONSULTATION, PATIENT ACCESS AND APPOINTMENT SYSTEMS

The encounter between patient and doctor is a core value in general practice.[2] Howie and colleagues describe two of these core values as 'patient-centredness' and 'holism'. The term 'patient-centred' first appeared in *The Future General Practitioner*, presented as an approach which encompasses 'the patient's total experience of illnesses', and it has come to represent the defining philosophy of general practice, emphasising the importance of taking patient beliefs and characteristics into consideration when making clinical decisions.[3] This contrasts with the disease-centred method in which only the doctor's agenda is addressed.[4] Consequently, this study enables us to see the two characteristics of this approach: patient-centred consulting and patient participation in decision making. This requires that the doctor facilitates the patient's expressing herself and that, for her part, the patient speaks openly and asks questions, and any conflict between doctor and patient should be settled by negotiation.[5]

Open Access

For patients, easy access to doctors at the surgery and at home carried a high level of priority. This was one of the main topics which troubled patients, and the patients interviewed were almost solidly against the introduction of appointments. The practice was one of the last in the area to adopt an appointment system, and many patients accepted the length of the wait for a particular doctor as an indication of the doctor's abilities. As we shall see, there were good arguments on both sides, and the medical literature shows benefits and drawbacks for the two methods.

However, change did come to the practice at the time that the interviews were being conducted. Most of the interviews were conducted before the full impact of the new appointment system, which began with appointments in the evening only, could be assessed. Patients were understanding that open doors until 6 p.m. meant that surgery sessions could extend well into the evening. Introduction of morning appointments came later.

The process of creating a relationship with a GP is an active, dynamic process. Patients want their doctor to take their symptoms seriously; to listen and/or ask questions about their symptoms; to treat them as a real person, not only as a patient; and to ask questions about other things than the disease, such as family or work issues. Access to the general practitioner and the problems related to appointment systems frequently came up in the interviews. Personal continuity of care was much prized by those interviewed, while factors like out-of-hours services, the growth of the practice with increasing numbers of doctors and the establishment of a multi-disciplinary practice team threatened the old images.[6] Patients began to differentiate between an acute consultation for a new self-limiting illness and the need to consult their regular doctor for ongoing and more chronic problems, which often had remissions and relapses.

In areas of high deprivation, such as Govan and Ibrox, the concentration of health and social problems within families and the concentration of such families within practices resulted in levels of need and demand which placed substantial and continuous pressures on primary health care teams. In such areas, primary care is often characterised by higher consultation rates, shorter consultation times and a larger list of problems to address within the consultation and GP's report limiting influences of time and stress.[7]

The open-access system meant that patients simply turned up at the designated times, usually between 9 a.m. and 11 a.m. and again between 4 p.m. and 6 p.m. from Monday to Friday but with a half day on Wednesdays. The surgery times had been inherited from pre-NHS days and allowed the doctors to catch up with house calls or practice administration or just to have a breather between the heavy toll of morning and afternoon consultations. Dr Ockrim had early afternoon surgeries on Tuesdays and Thursdays, aimed at children and pregnant women. There was also a surgery on Saturday mornings, officially for emergencies, open between 9 a.m. and 11 a.m. Before 1948, there was a surgery on Sunday mornings which was dropped before the National Health Service began.[8] The practice had inherited from Dr George the holding of a surgery late on Saturday afternoons. It was, supposedly, just for emergency consultations but was popular with patients who had been at the football match at the nearby Ibrox Stadium. It was only discontinued around 1958. The Saturday morning surgery continued until the deputising services, the Glasgow Emergency Medical Service (GEMS), provided full weekend cover. Sandra Grant, one of the receptionists, described the reception process at Cessnock Street:

> When the patients came in, they queued up at the window on the left-hand side. They gave their names and went in [to the waiting room] and waited for the doctor. They joined whatever queue and they just moved along the seats. As one went came out, the next one went in. We took their [record] cards out and we just slipped them into the doctor as a patient came out the room. We waited until there was a few and handed them in.

Patients understood that if they were prepared to wait to see their doctor that their doctor would wait to see them. Waiting times could be just a few minutes or be more than an hour, but a same-day consultation was guaranteed. A receptionist, Donalda MacQuarrie, recalled that at peak times, 'quite a lot of them were actually standing outside. The waiting rooms were actually full, and they had to stand in a corridor and out into the street because sometimes it was so busy'.

With open access, the practice was never in a situation of seeing patients being turned away or being offered fit-in slots by duty doctors or even locums. However, one problem with open access was that it was usually difficult for reception staff to persuade patients to see locum or trainee doctors, as other than for minor complaints, it always seemed best to consult a familiar doctor. We have seen that in the early days, many patients were wary of seeing a woman doctor. Just a few years later, that had changed significantly. As Dr Gordon had mentioned in his reference about her work in Blantyre, it was Dr Ockrim's skills—her knowledge, decisiveness and empathy—which very quickly made the difference. In addition, within a few years, there would have been many patients who had had a child, or a grandchild, delivered under her direction. Thus, prejudice was mitigated by consulting with the familiar: Dr Ockrim had become the tried and trusted doctor, unless, of course, patients were prepared to cross her when she counselled (men) about alcohol excess, spouse abuse and malingering.

Digby, writing in 1999, notes that 'discussion of the dynamics of the patient-doctor encounter is a feature of the recent past', indicating that studies of the encounter in earlier times had to be derived from a variety of other sources.[9] This underlines the importance of this oral history which explores this relationship with memories stretching back in some cases to the 1930s. These recollections augment much of what we know from such sources as the Women's Health Enquiry of 1933, featuring over a thousand working-class women.[10] The Enquiry showed that the women had a variety of options, besides a medical consultation, but that medical advice was sought more often by the more affluent of respondents.

The Black Report showed that the population most in need for primary health care may find that appointment systems act more as a barrier, with the receptionist placed between them and the doctor.[11] In other words, appointment systems facilitate the use of general practitioners by the more articulate while discouraging use among the socially deprived. In turn, this could further increase health inequalities. Given the situation of the practice in an area clearly recognised as showing high levels of deprivation, the absence of an appointments system was seen as facilitating access by the neediest parts of the community.

The senior partners, those who had joined the practice in the 1940s, had been loath to abandon open access. However, patients were able to see some of its problems. The rule was that the doors were open till 6 p.m., and someone arriving at 6:01 p.m. was liable to be disappointed. However, hard decisions and flexibility could cause their own problems, and even what seemed like a simple request at the reception window could upset patients.

I phoned for my heart pills and was told I would have to come along to the surgery. I said, 'I don't know if I can make it [in time]'. I got ready and when I got ready, I thought I could make it, so I came out and I got in here at about five to six. I got my turn to wait, and I sat outside for a wee while because sometimes there's a musty smell in there.[12] Anyway, I went back to tell the girl that any doctor would do me—it was only a prescription I was in for . . . the next thing the door goes, so the girl came round, and said, 'I'm sorry we're closed'. The man said, 'Oh, but darlin''—She lets him in full of drink. I thought, well that's a good one. I broke my neck to get along here for five to six and she lets two in who are worse for drink.

(DD)

I think your [entrance] hall is too small because on a cold, wet, windy day it's full of people. I have stood outside on an occasion when it was cold and wet. I know you can't make it like Hampden Park [but].

(FC)

Appointments

The move to the new premises in Midlock Street led to a re-opening of the debate about appointments, and it was eventually decided to start with evening appointments while leaving the mornings open for surgeries. It was clear, by the end of the 1980s, as Dr Ockrim was planning to retire, that the open-access system was no longer functioning for good practice in the evenings. The view from the office, as well as from the doctors, was quite clear. Doctors and staff had other commitments, families, child-care and work for the evening deputising services which had evening shifts which began at 6 p.m. Open access in the evening had become untenable. One of the receptionists, Sandra Grant, said that she welcomed the idea of evening appointments:

I think it is a good idea because the evening surgeries are becoming really long. Sometimes we weren't getting out until 8 o'clock at night. . . . With having open access in the morning, you are still giving a good service to people. They know they are going to be seen on the day that they want to be seen. It will take a bit of getting used to for the patients and for us, but I think it will work.

Another receptionist, Donalda MacQuarrie, agreed:

I actually think the patients have accepted it not too badly. . . . I think if they don't get the doctor that they want that day, I think they'll come to the morning surgery.

The introduction of evening appointments while maintaining open access in the mornings led to greater acceptance, or at least greater understanding, when morning appointments were eventually introduced not long after Dr Ockrim retired. She had been happy with the first-come-first-serve approach and was personally sorry to see it go. It has been pointed out that when urgent consultations were allocated to a duty doctor, which partners usually prefer, there is a loss of personal medical care.[13] Schers and colleagues wrote, based on patient surveys in the Netherlands, that in a changing society with apparent emphasis on turbulence and short-lived interpersonal contacts, most patients within general practice continue to value a personal doctor for serious and emotional problems, regardless of age, sex, place of residence and present circumstances. Also, patients appear to value personal continuity because they think that this will be beneficial to their health.[14]

While the personal physician is, as described by Jones and colleagues, the 'gold standard' for consultations, patients understood that there were, of necessity (illness, holidays, study leave), limits to availability.[15] Still, fifteen years after the interviews began, it was noted that there remained a dearth of evidence of improved clinical outcome related to open access as against appointments.[16] The open-access system allowed for varying times for consultations—the simple signing of a form might take just a couple of minutes, while a complex medical problem would take much longer. Morrell and colleagues saw no evidence for patients who attended for a five-minute appointment receiving more prescriptions, more hospital referrals or even repeat consultations within the next month.[17] While Howie and colleagues had found that there was more to patient outcomes, they also reported that more long-term health problems were recognised and that there was more time for health promotion, leading to greater patient satisfaction.[18]

The number of consultations at Cessnock Street was generally high, with doctors having to see thirty or more patients at some morning surgeries, allowing the patients just around five or six minutes with the doctor. Crowded surgeries and time constraints had a marked effect on the doctors in Cessnock Street. In the early days, consulting time had to include procedures, such as ear syringing, changing of dressings and blood tests which were later undertaken by practice nurses.

Patients were, therefore, appreciative that they could be seen when they wished to initiate contact with the doctor, and the receptionists only had to pass the case notes to the doctor. They knew that that their doctor would be aware of past history and all the other issues which could have an influence on the consultation. The problems that most patients found with appointments related to the perceived difficulty in accessing a quick medical assessment for an acute illness, though not all, felt the same way.

I think it was your words years ago—'If you want to see me, well I've other patients. If you want to see me, you'll wait for me'. You just cannae rush a doctor tae see you.

(LI)

I prefer seeing the doctor when I am ill. I think it is the height of nonsense that you should phone up a doctor and they say you can only have an appointment in two days-time. Two days can be an awfully long time if you are in pain or anxiety about something.

(IS)

You always had a long wait in the surgery before you were taken. We don't mind, we would rather have it that way than have an appointment. I never felt rushed. You didn't dally because you knew the doctors were busy.

(LN)

When I hear other people that have appointment systems with their doctors, they phone up and cannae get an appointment for a week or a fortnight—I think that's garbage. My husband has got an appointment system and I think it's terrible.

(YM)

I don't see the point in it. Is it to get more patients or what? I know there is quite a lot of them but that's what I like about our own surgery. If I don't feel really well one day I can go down and maybe see the doctor the next day. My neighbour upstairs—I had to phone for her wee boy on Monday and she wasn't getting taken until yesterday morning. I think that's terrible for a boy of ten. As I said to her, 'You should just call him out and tell him that you need to see him'.

(BE)

Personally, I would prefer an appointment system. I don't like sitting in a big waiting room with a lot of people and kids screaming around me. I don't like that very much. It wouldn't stop me. Well, I don't have to wait too long generally. I time it so that if I'm going to go there, I go in just before 11. I have always.

(ZT)

They [the doctors] are very helpful. They're no' there to get you in and push you out quick. They'll let you sit and tell them everything you want to tell them and they're very understanding. Great support. It doesnae matter if it takes you two minutes or twenty-two minutes, they'll sit and listen. I have been in twenty minutes before.

(DX)

Yes, you could see any doctor, that's why I liked it as well. You didn't have to make an appointment. If you felt ill, you just went over, and you could see any doctor that was available. Yes, there were enough chairs, but sometimes it was that busy, a few people had to stand, but usually they kept moving quite well. Sometimes it was very, very busy. Well, sometimes it was half an hour or three-quarters of an hour [waiting to see the doctor], it just depended.

(ITt)

Ron Campbell, a former senior porter at the Southern General Hospital, who was well aware of how GP surgeries functioned, commented:

What I remember of the practice at Cessnock Street—I used to always think it was like Argyle Street[19] when you went in, because there was no appointment system, which I admire. I don't agree with appointment systems, because I think at the end of the day appointment systems don't always work. I believe in the first come first serve.

As the doctor knew the patient, their life story and extensive family connections, some surgery visits were very brief if all that was required was a form be signed, such as confirmation of an illness. Other consultations took whatever time was required, and there was an understanding that these longer encounters were an essential part of the doctor–patient relationship. However, there was a sense that this relationship was beginning to change:

I actually preferred the old doctors. The new ones, I suppose, will be ok but it takes a bit of getting used to. You got to know the doctors and they were friends as well as being your doctor and if you had any problems, you knew you could go to them. I think you felt closer to the doctors before. . . when you are getting on in years it may be you feel you would like a doctor to be a wee bit older.

(ITt)

The Waiting Room

The crowded waiting room functioned as a social centre and was highly valued by many. For some patients who had been relocated to the peripheral housing schemes, it also offered an opportunity to visit the old areas and perhaps meet up with former neighbours, friends and family.

> I thought it was very good. It always did and yet people'll say—I'll say I was doon at the doctors at Ibrox. 'Whit dae ye go away tae Ibrox for when there's doctors roon' here?' I say, 'It's just like a family, you're used to it, so you don't want to change.' If the doctors had said change, we would change but they were quite willin' tae take us. It's just noo, we're usin' the doctors more than ever. I think it's very good.
>
> (IO)

Elizabeth Whyteman recalled the following:

> It was a good way of meeting your family. We all went down to the surgery, and we all met there. We all knew where one another was. It was a family practice. I think it was nice. It was very close knit. I liked it anyway. Oh, I talk to a lot of people [in the Waiting Room]. I don't go in and just sit and look about me. Before you know it, you're busy blethering and talking away. I think it's nice. Before we know it, we see one another again. That's how you get to meet people. Aye it's nice and friendly. You go down there for a day out.
> Oh aye [I talk to people in the waiting room]. They'll talk about the doctors. They'll say, 'He's awful good or he's awful nice or I don't like her—Him, I wouldnae send my dog to him.' This is the sort of thing they say. Only because they probably didnae get the prescription they really wanted the time before. They'll maybe give you their life history, you know—from the day they were born till they came to this particular appointment. . . . A blether and a wee bit of company.
>
> (RN)

> I think it's very inviting now. It hasn't got the atmosphere of the smaller place [Cessnock] but that happens in everything in life. . . . I like it very much.
>
> (LN)

Some patients who had chronic health problems themselves were often surprised to be given the details of their neighbours' medical issues in the waiting room.

> Yes, you talk [in the waiting room]. People who are there waiting tell you their problems and then you wonder why you're there.
>
> (DT)

Linda McMahon noted that receptionists were often trying to quieten bored children in the waiting room, which at busy times could be very noisy. The staff were concerned that some children might leave toys on the floor, which could be a hazard for elderly patients. She commented:

> They used to be terribly hard on children [in the Waiting Room]—I noticed that. There was nothing for children to do, no area where they could sit and play with toys or look at books or draw, and yet the staff seemed to think they should sit quietly. I always went provided with books for the children, but not everyone thinks of that.

Another patient remarked:

> I've never really had any thoughts at all to put in the suggestion box, but [my son] has, but we didn't put it in. He wants something to play with while he's waiting. [I have seen] a couple of children maybe squabbling about something or running around making a loud noise but nothing other than that.
>
> (KN)

Dr Ockrim was aware of this and thought that she might give a gift to the practice on her retirement of some child-friendly toys. Smaller toys provided in the past quickly disappeared, so she recalled the following:

> When I left, I suggested giving them a trampoline or a chute or something and the office staff just about went mad when I suggested it.

However, a children's play table soon appeared:

> I like the way they've got that wee table for the kids now. The other week I was there, there was two wee ones and did they enjoy it! It was nice watching them.
>
> (ISo)

The experience of these interviews is that patients generally did not feel hurried and that due attention was paid to their concerns and individual needs. When appointments were introduced at Midlock, patients were allocated ten minutes, almost double the average time of an open-access consultation, and this alone may have helped anchor the new system. However, this meant that the new system could not offer the same number of consultations as had been available under open access. Offering repeat prescriptions at longer intervals helped save appointment slots, but patients who expected to meet family and friends in the waiting room followed by a supportive chat with the doctor, without any fresh medical issues to discuss, were likely to be disappointed.

CONSULTATION CONTENT

It was said that, too easy, contacts with the doctor could come at a price on the practitioner's health, with the stress of having a heavy workload and dealing with the NHS bureaucracy.[20] The consultation and the doctor's caring attitude produced an undeniable placebo effect, and every consultation was expected to conclude with a prescription.[21] Doctors could feel rushed, and patients could feel frustrated by lengthy waits. In later years, given the open access in the evening surgeries, the numbers entering before the doors closed at 6 p.m. could take an hour or more to clear.

There's no' been a time when I needed a doctor or needed to go to the surgery or anything like that—there was always somebody there—and there's always an ear to listen to you. You always have somebody there that's interested in your welfare. I think so. I could always discuss it with you . . . when I was young and I came to you and I had any problems, If I didnae tell you, my auntie did. I never was embarrassed, because in my opinion, you were the person that could help. If anything was wrong and it could be put right, you could help to do that.

(INa)

Because you could just go doon there at 8 o' clock in the morning and sit and wait for you coming in. It's not the same as it used tae be. I'll go doon when I need my pills, and that's it. I sometimes don't even go doon. I used to love going doon tae the surgery and it was homely. . . . I used tae come oot after I had spoke to you for an hour and I felt brilliant all day.

(LD)

I was always concerned [at the surgery] that I didn't catch anything that would keep me off my work and everyone spluttering around me.

(ZI)

Some doctors, even in thae days, had ideas of grandeur—They were doctors you know, *bow doon* or *salaam me* or whatever. That was their idea of being a doctor but as I say, they were above what they were able to perform because it was a' in their mind. If you went into your surgery and explained 'what was the matter?'—'Nothing's too much bother. I'll try and get something to fix that.'

(INa)

I consider myself to be very friendly with Dr David and he was a kind of father figure to me, and I had no closeness between me and my [own] father. When there were difficulties in my life, adolescence or whatever, I found David Collins was a great listener. I would take up half an hour of his time. I'm sure many others as well did. If I was having a low—I would make up some kind of physical condition and go along and see about it. I didn't go along and say I wanted a chat, but I got a chat out of it. So, he was very special in my life.

(ZT)

Oh aye. I found that the doctor always spends the time with the patient that would satisfy himself and his diagnosis. I've never found anything else in our surgery. That's always been the pattern in our surgery. If you needed a certain examination to diagnose, you got it and there was always a very thorough— Dr Collins Senior was tremendous. Many a time when I've gone in with my skin in such a state, he would take the time to look at it. He wouldnae just say, oh here's tablets—He would take the time and look at it and say, we'll try this and that. . . . Many a time I was all bandaged up and he would take the time to help me off with it and look at it and put a fresh bandage on.

(QD)

I've heard them saying, 'You go in there and you're oot before you're in and I don't know how they know whit's rang wi' me. They're writing lines out before you get sitting down.' I've never found that. Even when I was working, if I went down because I had the flu or something, I was wanting something for it, there was never a case of you sitting writing a line out before I even got in. I don't know where they get it from. Some people just find something to complain about. If they wernae complainin' they wouldnae be happy.

(HNi)

Ronald Campbell was not shy in warning me if he knew that a patient, who was on his staff of porters at the Southern General, was malingering, 'swinging the boot' as he put it:

I remember once in the hospital I had one of my staff who was a patient of the practice, and I knew he was swinging the boot a wee bit, so I phoned and one time I was in seeing Dr Kenneth. I said, 'I think this fellow is swinging the boot a wee bit and I told him some of the things this fellow was up to outside.' Then, I had that relationship with the doctor that I could do that. He was obviously conning the doctor a wee bit.

Elizabeth Temple, who had been the local chemist, was aware of changes in consultation outcomes, as doctors were increasingly prescribing pre-packaged items:

When we started first of all there was a lot of the British National Formula. We made up more actual prescriptions and there was less sophistication in the drugs of course. Gradually it became that you were just counting out tablets and filling up bottles and putting on labels.

However, patients arriving at the reception window often wanted something other than a consultation with the doctor. It could be information on any of the practice services, and the following shows that patients could be frustrated by the rule that receptionists were not allowed to disclose medical information about family members without written permission:

I never found the clerical staff very friendly or co-operative. I think they are dreadful. I think their attitude—there was a wee lassie on yesterday and I gave my name clear and gave my [practice] number. My wife had asked if I would get her cholesterol result and it was as if I was asking for a fish supper. When I go into a shop and get that kind of response it upsets me too. I think that if they are there and you are paying them good money, they should have some kind of rapport. They are not there for pleasure.

(FC)

The position of the practice receptionist in the busy office, standing at the window and receiving dozens of patients in an incredibly short time, inevitably led to tensions, not all of which were capable of easy resolution. With the absence of appointments and patients being seen on a first-come-first-seen basis, there could often be exceptionally busy periods and other times which were much quieter. Most patients seemed happy to accept the possibility of a long wait when they knew that they could be seen at a time of their choosing.

WORKING PRACTICES

From the beginning, the office staff had clearly delineated tasks to perform. While the procedures were relatively straightforward, the atmosphere was often quite frenetic. Without an appointment system, the patient's records could not be located in advance which might have freed staff time to deal with paperwork, sort out forms, and make and receive phone calls.

Two of the receptionists described the problems which could occur in the reception area.

> I think you just get a bit tired talking the whole day to patients and you always get your arguments and things that they didn't agree with. The first person they see is you, so you get the brunt of anything that goes wrong. We don't take prescriptions over the phone, and we would tell a patient that and they would say it was a lot of rubbish because the doctor had told them to phone and things like that. They thought we were being obstructive some of the time and I think wires get crossed sometimes.
>
> (Donalda MacQuarrie, Receptionist)

While drunks were a frequent occurrence, violent incidents were fortunately rare but seemed to increase in the new premises. Nanette Aitken described one event at Midlock Street: 'That was the first encounter of anything going wrong. Here it's an every-day occurrence'. She recalled an incident at Cessnock Street:

> When I started, I think I came across one drunk man that was really abusive. He came out—he went into Dr Collins, and he just wouldn't take no for an answer. We tried to be diplomatic with him, but he just came out and slammed the doctor's door and came into the reception area and it was a glass door, and he slammed the door and the door just shattered.

In another, more frightening event in Midlock Street, Nanette described the events when a female patient under the influence of drink or drugs was described as 'rather abusive', and when challenged, she did the following:

> produced the shaft of a hammer from her sleeve . . . started wielding this and she hit the brand-new pillars, which annoyed me and hit the brand-new seats and then fortunately the trainee came to my assistance. By this time, the receptionist had phoned the police and she was apprehended.

The increase in the size of the staff and the need to form good working relationships led to regular joint social as well as training events. Nanette Aitken explained:

> Over the years we have developed some nights out and this includes the doctors, and we go to bowling nights. We are all on first name terms which is very good. It is more of a complete team rather than having bosses and staff. We also have a Christmas dinner evening which has been very successful, and they can all let their hair down. I think the working conditions are very good.

The new contract in 1965/1966 brought about many changes in the office. With access by GPs to hospital laboratory services, there were the results of blood and urine tests to be filed. Copies of referral letters to the hospital, replies from outpatients and the hospital discharge letters also had to be filed, and extra office shelving was needed as case folders expanded. Increased health service bureaucracy required extra form filling which in turn led to the need for more staff to process them. Before computerisation, which simplified the system, there were forms for ordering forms for ordering forms.

> I think the paperwork [now] takes up all of the time. I'm doing more paperwork [related to practice accounts and item of service claim forms] now than I have ever done.
>
> (Donalda MacQuarrie)

CONSULTING A WOMAN DOCTOR

We have noted the history of women in medicine and their increasing presence in general practice. However, 'entrenched' attitudes, as one participant put it, took some time to change. Becoming a full-time partner in general practice in 1946 did not mean that the prejudices against women doctors in the past were over. Dr Ockrim had to encounter many challenges within the practice until the patients were used to her and the role of a woman doctor. The following shows a range of views on the role of women doctors as they saw it in their own practice.

> I feel I cannae talk to a man. I missed you terrible when you went. Tae me you're no a doctor, tae me you're my friend as well as a doctor.
>
> (LD)

This patient refused to change her doctor when she moved outside the practice area, indicating her discomfort at the idea of starting to build a new relationship in a different practice:

> I've known you since I was a wee lassie. It's a' right for him to say you've flitted; you'll need to change your doctors. I could come and talk to you and tell you all my problems.
>
> (5LD)

I was with [a male doctor] and he told me I was pregnant, so I came over to your practice because I preferred a lady doctor.

(ITa)

However, this was not a universal attitude, and certainly, in the late 1940s and early 1950s, there remained serious prejudice against women in medicine. This had already existed during Dr Stevan George's time, but these attitudes clearly persisted after the practice changeover in 1946:

The entrenched thought of people those days, nobody wanted to go to the lady doctor and there was always a big queue for Dr George.

(AS)

I think in the old days very few people went to see you because you were a lady doctor. My son-in-law always used to go to you, and they would say, 'Look at that jessie sittin' there to go to Dr Ockrim'.

(CT)

One patient described how her husband, complaining of chest pain, preferred to go home without seeing a female doctor, with disastrous consequences. While it would be impossible to apportion blame for a fatal outcome in an illness where sudden death often occurs, the story resonates with the grief and anger of the bereaved wife.

When I came out the hospital, I came down to see you and my husband was with me and I said to you that—and the receptionist took me in without waiting and I went in to you and I said to you and you said, 'Oh, you're fine' and I said 'Yes'. I said, 'My husband's outside, he's been complaining of chest pain'. You said, 'Tell him to wait and see one of the other doctors'. So, when I came out, I said to him, 'Come and we'll see one of the other doctors'.

He wouldn't come in with me because you were a woman doctor. I said, 'Why don't we wait and see? He said, 'No, no we'll just go home'. After he died—he was actually dead—he just dropped dead. When they phoned [the surgery] and told the [male] doctor, he came out to the house and he was chalk white and I stood, and I bawled and shouted at him.

(BC)

In fact, in the early days, it was not unusual for most patients to choose to see the male doctor. A couple of patients recalled the following incident, which occurred in the early 1950s, some decades before the practice introduced an appointments system, and waiting times were often long:

I was sitting with the children in the big waiting room and there was a big queue. So, they were all waiting for Dr Collins at this side, and the next thing Dr Ockrim flares out of her room, stands with her hands on her hips, and says, 'I'm a doctor too, you know—NEXT!' Everyone just sat with their mouths open and there was a few laughs. She was quite right.

(IH)

The other recollection of the same, or perhaps a similar, incident focusses on Dr Ockrim's intolerance of malingerers. Someone wanting some time off work for a medical condition which could not be proved objectively, such as backache, would hardly be likely to consult her.

> I remember just one time. You were to blame. They were all waitin' to get in for Dr Collins and you were in that wee side room and you says, 'Next, please!' I was waitin' on someone movin' and naebody moved and you came out and you said, 'Right,' to this man. You said, 'Oh aye, just wait for him, he gives the sick lines out'—and you shouted and bawled at him. I said to myself, 'Oh.' You didn't give the sick lines.[22] Aye, you knew a' their faces. I'll never forget that day. This man says, 'Look at the size o' her tae.'

(IO)

During the 1970s, there was a significant influx into the area of patients from Pakistan and India that had a more conservative attitude to gender issues and who actively sought out a practice with a woman doctor. If no female doctor was available, a family member always accompanied the female patient:

> my mum went to Dr Ockrim, because she was a female. It is in our religion. We always went to a female rather than a male doctor. A male always went to a male.

(HC)

An abused woman commented:

> I used to always have to talk to a man doctor. I don't know. I think I was more dominated by a male. I reckon that's the answer. Mostly, because it's been a male that's dominated you all your life. I don't know why that happens. I think it goes back to your mother. She didnae help so you didnae feel she was interested. You felt that women were just a waste of time.

(DM)

This patient did, however, come to consult with Dr Ockrim, able to see in a woman of authority a sense of the ability to control that had been lacking in her own life:

> When I was a kid, you gave me the impression that you didnae like ma da' and I liked that. I felt you had more power over him, but at the same time I couldn't talk to you about it.
> Aye, I felt kind of close, but no' close enough to tell you [about the abuse]. There was something powerful about you that I liked. There was a lot of

people didnae like you. I used to say to people, 'She's straight forward and she'll tell you to your face what she thinks.' There was just something aboot you. My da' was always with me. You used to say to my da'—'Are you still drinking? Do you not think it's about time you stopped drinking?' You were saying this, and I thought, that's great. My ma couldnae dae that and I used tae see you stronger than my da'.

(DM)

Some testimony from this participant, who had suffered physical and sexual abuse from her father, will be discussed in the next chapter.

PRACTICE STAFF

The growth in the employed practice staff in Cessnock Street and subsequently in Midlock Street mirrored developments nationally.[23] Bosanquet and Salisbury trace the development of *General Practice under the National Health Service* from 1948 to 1990. They describe the introduction of partial reimbursement of staff salaries, from the landmark 1965 GP contract. This helped provide the resources to recruit the receptionists and others needed to manage the practice and to forge a relationship with the central administration of general practitioners in Glasgow. This administration was done, firstly, through the local Executive Council and, later, with the Primary Care Services of the Greater Glasgow Health Board. The areas served by Executive Councils were designed to serve a particular area but did not necessarily have the same boundaries as the medical services retained by local authorities.[24] With payments based on capitation and item of service, there was a constant flow of forms from practices to the Executive Council.

The first receptionists appeared in Cessnock Street almost from the start of the arrival of Drs David and Ockrim. Someone was needed to welcome patients, take their details and provide the doctor with their record envelopes. Nanette Aitken, later practice manager, started working at Cessnock Street on 28th August 1966, when the medical staff consisted of three full-time doctors and a part-time assistant. Despite the size of the practice, which stabilised around 9,000 patients from the 1950s, the practice functioned with just one office worker until 1976. Gradually, the role of the office workers expanded, and the concept of a practice manager emerged.[25] In 1978, Donalda MacQuarrie joined the office staff, and by the time Sandra Grant arrived in 1981, Nanette had been appointed as a practice manager, and three others were working as receptionists or general office staff.

When Joan Kilcullen joined the reception staff in 1989, there were six whole-time equivalent (WTE) doctors, three practice nurses, in addition to the two attached district nurses and two health visitors. There was also a part-time dietician and a nurse working on a specific research project related to incontinence in the community. Changes in patient registration requirements made it easier for patients to change doctors.

Oh yes. We are getting a lot more, new patients now that it's easier for them to change their doctor. You find that you get a lot more coming in and going.

Moving into the area and staying in flats and then moving on. So, they are changing all the time. Yes, [there is a big turn over] especially with the young ones. The young ones only tend to stay a year and then move on, and they change their GP all the time. By the time we process them and get their old records in, that's only a couple of weeks and they are going elsewhere, and their records are going back again. It's causing a lot of work for us to get them all sorted out to the way we like them and then passing them on to another GP.

(Joan Kilcullen)

[The nurses do the] smears, blood pressure. The nurses actually do a lot of asthma clinics, hypertension clinics. There's a lot of [health promotion] clinics now that never was in Cessnock Street. It tends to be the nurses that are doing these.

(Nanette Aitken, Practice Manager)

SURGERY PREMISES

In the first years of the NHS, little changed in the layout of the surgery premises. The introduction of the Family Doctor Charter, with its encouragement of improvements in GP surgeries, opened the way for major changes. The development of the surgery premises can be seen in the context of wider provision for improved primary care facilities. Until 1966, the Cessnock Street Surgery consisted of two proper consulting rooms and one interview room, that is without an examination couch. The interview room was just used, as we have noted, on a Monday night when all the partners consulted at the same time. Reducing the size of the main waiting room enabled the interview room to be converted into a full-sized consulting room. Space was then taken from the caretaker's accommodation to provide an extra consulting room and some extra waiting space.

In 1980, with the death of the caretaker, two extra rooms were added to the surgery. These both became additional consulting rooms. Dr Ockrim's former room became a full-sized office space which could accommodate additional clerical staff and the extra shelving needed for A4-sized record folders. The small space, formerly used by the practice receptionist, became a base for NHS-employed attached nurses and health visitors. There was also a consulting room for Dr Barry Adams-Strump, who had arrived as a new partner in 1979, after working for a few months as a locum for Dr David Collins, who had suffered a stroke which eventually necessitated his retiral. Until 1978, when Dr David retired, only two doctors consulted in the surgery in the morning, while the two most junior doctors were out of the surgery dealing with the heavy load of house calls. This involved them covering a practice area which stretched from Ibrox in all directions, reaching Pollok, Nitshill, Croftfoot, Castlemilk and even Newton Mearns. Gradually, the load of house calls diminished and from 1978, when Dr David retired, three doctors consulted at the surgery in the morning, and only one doctor was out on house calls.

At Cessnock Street, there was no space for a treatment room, as all the rooms were needed for the doctors or were waiting rooms or office space. Blood and urine tests, injections and treatments, like bandaging and dressings, were all done by the doctor which obviously imposed constraints on consulting time. Donalda Mac-Quarrie remembered:

> There was no accommodation [for the practice staff] at all. It was just the reception area which was actually a glorified long corridor. . . . We had the files on one side and a window and a typewriter at the other.

The practice manager, Nanette Aitken, recalled that she worked alone for her first ten years in the practice, expected to do all the tasks required:

> [I did] everything. When I first started the patients would come in and I wouldn't be able to find records for them because we didn't have records for some of the patients. They would insist that they had been patients for years and years and that they should have records. I contacted the Health Board and we arranged that I would go up in an afternoon and type lists of all our patients and then compare them with the records we already had. We got the records straight and the patients would come in and give their name at the window and I would look out the cards for them and I would put them in to the doctors. I would file the cards at the end, answer the phone, take dictation, type letters, make coffee, go for the biscuits and any other odd job that would occur. . . .
>
> When I first started, I had contact with the patients from [when] they came through the door until they left, and everything connected with them. Repeat prescriptions were done on demand at the desk and not as they are today. As the staff increased, I did less work at the reception desk and did more of the clerical and typing.

By 1986, it was clear that the surgery would have to leave Cessnock Street. The City Council that owned the building planned to refurbish it, and it was made clear that there would be no room for commercial property which is what the authorities considered a medical practice to be. The search then began to find alternative premises, and fortunately, a site, in Midlock Street, belonging to the City of Glasgow, was identified just three streets away. Along with consulting rooms for all the doctors, including trainee practitioners, there would be improved office space, patient areas, treatment rooms and bases for district nurses and health visitors. There was also space for practice meetings, a small practice library and rooms for occasional sessions for a dietician and social worker. Soon, additional space was needed for the practice nurses. A substantial extension took care of all these requirements, funded by a mixture of NHS grants and practice loans.

The new practice building, the Midlock Medical Centre, opened in February 1987.

> We had to do [the move from Cessnock to Midlock] it over a weekend. We finished [at Cessnock] on the Saturday morning and immediately started to move which meant that we had to have the patients' records taken from Cessnock and installed in Midlock Street, in the right order. We are talking

about 9,000 plus, patient records. We had the equipment which was being moved—all in a matter of a day and a half. We ferried it back and forward with a hired van. The doctors, receptionists, sons, husbands, boyfriends—everybody mucked in. It was good fun, and it was hard work. Actually, everybody enjoyed it.

(Nanette Aitken)

Inevitably, comparisons were made with Cessnock Street. Everyone understood that the facilities were much superior and more comfortable for the patients, but the new developments came at a price, as a break from the past often does. Cessnock was seen by patients and staff to be 'warm and homely', even as conditions deteriorated in its last months, while Midlock was 'clean and clinical'. Donalda MacQuarrie explained her fondness for what had been left behind:

When I started at Cessnock Street I used to think, 'What have I got here?' but looking back now, I would go back to Cessnock Street tomorrow, no hesitation at all. I feel there was more companionship. I felt there was more friendliness. It's too big an area now and you just don't get to know the people. It's just passing talk. There is no intimate conversation. I just think it's a big surgery and unless you are actually with the girls you are actually working with—you know them very well, and I get on well with them, but I don't know the health visitors or the nurses. You don't get to know their personal side of life. In Cessnock Street everybody knew everybody. . . . I even feel as if I don't know half the people that work here. . . . When I started at first there was only Nanette and I. . . . We coped really well. The filing at night was done before we went away. We were never really very late. Quarter past six was a late night.

The surgery was the last tenant to leave before the building work began, and the last winter in Cessnock Street was particularly uncomfortable, as Donalda MacQuarrie recalled the following:

I can remember during the [last] winter at Cessnock Street when we used to have to come in with our wellies and keep our raincoats on, because the water was pouring through the ceiling, and we had to put [a] tarpaulin down in Dr Ockrim's room. We had fungus growing out the toilets because it was so damp in some of the rooms. We had to make holes in the ceiling sometimes to let the water come in. That was just before we moved. The building above was empty and I think people had stolen slates from the roof and the water was pouring in upstairs and there was something like two tons of water above us and it was slowly making its way down to us.

Well, we have a very much enlarged office area, and our record system is expanding. We have, at the moment, enough room for them as they are, but we are still having to put more shelves in to cope, which we couldn't possibly have done at Cessnock Street. The most important one that I found was the A4 folders. That was the thing. When we came along here, and we had them all out it really looked very impressive. We thought at the time we had plenty of room, but we are running out of room again. Space was a thing we saw the biggest difference in. There was plenty of room and you weren't tripping over yourself, and you had some place to sit down.

(Donalda MacQuarrie)

This last comment is somewhat ironic. When the surgery was being planned in late 1985, it was reckoned that there might need to be space for one office computer and that practice record folders would require increasing amounts of room. By 2020, there were computer terminals everywhere, patient records were accessed electronically and the folders were stored out of the office.

It was not long before there were examples of petty vandalism around the new surgery. The low roof encouraged children to climb around the roof tiles, but the main problems were inside the building and the car park.

We used to have soap dispensers on the wall [of the toilets] and they actually set that on fire, and it set the alarm off. They smoke in the toilets. They are beginning to write on the walls outside. They burn the bells off the door. It's just wanton vandalism. They stick chewing gum on the carpets.

(Donalda MacQuarrie)

Initially there was a lot of vandalism. The children created a great deal of problems in the summer. They still do, to a certain extent. I like the winter, because they are not around in the winter. The roof in this building is very low and are able to get onto the roof and cause quite considerable damage. Really from the word go, we've had broken windows and we've had the instance where they put super glue in the locks. Fortunately, we were inside, because if we had been outside, we would never have got [back] inside. We had to get the locksmith out to renew the locks.

(Nanette Aitken)

Practice Records

In 1980–1981, work began on changing the patient record system from the outdated Lloyd George envelopes, always referred to as cards, to the more familiar A4 folder, as used in hospitals. While practices in England had to pay for the better record format, the Scottish NHS covered the costs of the materials, and it was just left to the individual practices to make the arrangements for the changeover.[26] The new A4 records were to be eventually replaced by computerised records, but at the time of the move to Midlock Street in 1987, ample space was given to the A4 records which needed much more shelving than the small envelopes they replaced. The task of moving the notes from the record envelopes to the new folders was complex and time-consuming.

Yes. I had just started in the Practice at that time, and I got the job of sticking on all the sticky labels on to the cards. I remember that well. I remember us coming along with all the boxes of cards—it was a big job, and it took a long time for the complete change-over of the card system. The system that we have today is great.

It [the new GP Contract] has certainly made more paperwork but as for the standard of health care, I have my doubts about that. There is so much paperwork to do now and so many other things. Instead of just concentrating on getting a patient better now, you've got to go through all these papers and find out if you are doing the right thing. Everything you do now, there's a paper attached to it. Your mind is taken up with that more than actually getting patients well or getting them to attend.

(Sandra Grant)

HOUSE CALLS AND DOMICILIARY VISITS

An important part of general practice has been the doctor attending the patient at home when required. When the National Health Service began, it was estimated that around 25–33% of consultations took place in the patient's home, though the proportion began to fall with time.[27] There were many reasons for the doctor carrying out a house call. There was a reluctance to move sick patients, especially with an acute illness, from home to the surgery, especially if they lived at the far end of the catchment area in areas such as Darnley and Castlemilk. Many patients did not have access to a car, and mothers were often reluctant to bring a sick child to the surgery if it meant a two-bus journey. Others were concerned that the busy waiting room would be the breeding ground for infections. It was expected that fevered children would be seen at home, as would patients with chronic disabling illnesses. Many patients did not have a phone at home, and house call requests might be made by a neighbour or a relative, who often had limited information.

The GP contract states that the decision to make a house call is in the hands of the GP.[28] Mitchell et al. have recently pointed, in a post-Covid world, to a lack of a robust evidence base regarding GP home visits and relatively little research to understand the circumstances in which patients request GP home visits, when and why GPs undertake home visits and how outcomes can be optimised within a resource-constrained health service.[29]

In an entry on 'house calls' in Wikipedia, the steep decline on this form of doctor–patient encounter was noted in the United States, falling from around 40% of primary care consultations in the 1930s to less than 1% by 1980.[30] Studies from many different parts of Europe and North America have confirmed this trend. In general, British general practitioners have shown themselves to be aware of the role of house calls and their advantage in enabling comprehensive patient care. However, problems of the time involved and scarcity of facilities in the patient's home often militated against the concept.[31] Consequently, there have been calls recently for home visits in primary care to be delegated to an alternative health care professional.[32]

Data from consultation and house visit lists between 1989 and 1992 show that house calls in the practice were a little less than 10% of patient contacts, thus still forming an important part of doctor time, though much lower than the contacts made a generation earlier. Some of the testimony confirmed that house calls could be done for social as well as medical reasons, and the practice had a permissive attitude to accepting them, though in recent years there has been more of an attempt to triage requests. In 1973, a study was carried out at the Woodside Health Centre and the Glasgow University Department of General Practice which showed that only about one-third of the requested house calls were considered by the doctor to justify a visit, and some of these could have been seen the next day.[33] Of the remainder, most could have been either brought to the surgery that morning or advised to attend the evening surgery. The remaining quarter could have been treated by reassurance. The issues went beyond the elderly, chronically sick and housebound, and extended to many of the acutely ill, judged as unfit to attend at the surgery.

However, the good old days when the doctor had a much smaller array of medications and care was represented by the time spent at the bedside was recalled as follows:

> I think at the beginning she would be [kept in bed]. I wasn't born [yet] . . . but I do recall [hearing] that Dr Collins gave her every attention because what I remember is during the night even, no matter what time of the night or early morning, Dr Collins would come out. I can't remember if it would be an injection or tablets or whatever but whatever he would give her, he would come through to the kitchen and he said he wanted to wait and see what the reaction was. He would sit and have a cup of coffee and after a certain time he would leave. Now, that happened not just once or twice but over the years.
>
> (LM)

> Q. Why didn't you call the doctor if you felt so bad?
> A. I don't like to annoy the doctor coming to my house.
>
> Q. Do you think the doctor would mind?
> A. No, but I think he might be needed somewhere else.
>
> (DT)

> There was nobody like Dr [David] Collins. I don't think there ever will be. You see, when you wanted Dr Collins, Dr Collins came out. He didn't say, 'I can't make it, I'll send somebody else.' He just came out.
>
> (FS)

> This night I had went out with my husband. On the way home, I was quite sick. I said, 'I'll no' bother wi' the doctor' and I went into my bed. I was in my bed, and I was getting worse. I said, 'I think you better go and get the doctor.' He ran away down the street and phoned. Dr Collins came to the door. . . . He came in and he said I had pleurisy. He told my husband to—every four hours to waken me and give me these tablets during the night. By the morning my temperature had gone down. I said to Dr Collins, 'I'm awful sorry to get you out of bed'. He was there with his pyjamas under his jacket. He was actually in his pyjama jacket. He said to my husband, 'I knew when [you] phoned it was

something serious. He was so good'. He had a lovely bed-side manner.

(BC)

I remember, years ago, when [she] was a baby she suffered from severe ear-ache, and I remember having seen a child with mastoid, and I thought this was a possibility. I phoned your home, and you were out. However, someone got in touch with you and Dr Collins phoned out a prescription to an all-night chemist. We got the prescription and gave it to [her]. It was coming up to midnight when there was a knock at the door, and who was standing on the doorstep but Dr [David] Collins. Dr Collins came in and said that he was just passing. He said that I sounded quite worried about the baby's ear, and he thought that he would come in and have a wee look. You don't forget these things.

(DK)

I always remember Dr Russell—he would come, and we would say—we never sent for you. He said, I know but your mother was bad, this morning so I thought I would come up and see her. You don't get doctors doing that now.

(QD)

We have already noted the comments of ZI about the doctors' strong point being their bedside manner. He recalled the following:

I remember as a small boy, when one of the doctors would come to me if I had the flu. We were very impressed if they would sit there and talk to you and then you ended up with a bottle of some kind, which had great properties, according to the doctor, and it made you better.

(ZI)

Some patient recollections covered especially memorable house calls. Being able to deal with illness with a house-bound patient enabled the development of a particularly close bond between patient and doctor. I remember that on one occasion, a patient with cancer was refusing the hospital admission that Dr Ockrim had said was essential, and Dr Ockrim asked the patient what it would take for her to agree to the admission. The patient immediately said that she would like the dress the doctor was wearing when she had finished with it. Dr Ockrim had the dress cleaned, and it was waiting for the patient when she returned home. An important aspect of the doctor visiting the patient's home has been for supervising terminal care, considered in the chapter which includes cancer, but in other cases, it was assessing the situation regarding the need for home treatment or admission to hospital.

I collapsed in the shop [in 1949] and young Dr Russell, who had just joined your practice, someone had rushed across and got him. Dr Russell came across in a big hurry and he was greatly alarmed by my situation, and he helped me into his car and rushed me off to the Southern General. In the car I was vomiting, but I managed to open the door. I was concerned about his upholstery.

(ZI)

I remember my next-door neighbour and she came running into me one day and she said, 'Oh my god . . . oor [man] has just took a heart attack and we phoned the doctor and the doctor'll no' come oot.' I said, 'Wait and I'll give you the number o' oor surgery and phone them and explain what's happened and maybe some o' them'll come oot.' That's what happened—Dr Russell went oot. The man had came in from his work, took a heart attack sitting in the chair and died. He was only 46 and he had never been ill, never had an illness, it just came out of the blue and they couldnae get their own doctor to come.

(INa)

The practice was a long-time user of deputising services, though covering its own patients on the weekday evenings until midnight. It was only after this project was completed that in 1996, the service was reformed as the Glasgow Emergency Medical Service (GEMS). Some eight years later, the service was taken over by the NHS. As time went by, it was clear that there were risks in visiting some of the areas in the practice after surgery hours. Many of the requests for house calls were being made by addicts hoping that an unknown out-of-hours doctor might be more receptive to their request for opiates or that they might steal the doctor's medical bag. Ron Campbell related the following, based on his experience as a driver for the deputising service. It should be remembered that when the practice covered its evening calls, there was no driver to call for help in an emergency. Furthermore, the daily workload made the idea of a night on call an unwelcome prospect.

I had three arrested in Castlemilk one night. No, in the landing of the high flats. They were waiting for the doctor coming up. What they do is they phone for a doctor for such and such but it's actually not a genuine call. It's a hoax call, so that they can see the doctor coming and get the drugs. How is the controller to know it's a hoax call until you get there? The doctors' deputising service meets a need, but I still think a doctor from the practice is more important—if it's got sufficient doctors to do one night a week. Oh aye, in your young day as a doctor, you wouldnae have given it a thought . . . but if it was now, you would have second thoughts about going into certain areas. Even to your own people in your own practice.

(Ron Campbell)

[This] is the best surgery to put a call in without having them nagging at you. I know other people in other surgeries and their doctor is always moaning and groaning over them coming out to the house. I've found that [this] surgery is excellent for calling people out.

(FC)

I think there was one doctor who went up to my aunt and was a bit snappy and that upset her. [The] doctor told her she should come down to the surgery and get her prescription. My aunt put her in her place, but I also attended to that.

(QD)

I think that was the first time you had ever came up to the house 'cause I always went tae the surgery. I only called out the doctor when I really needed it. Aye, I was used tae you and I didnae like phonin' somebody oot 'cause I knew it was somebody else that was gonnae come.

(LD)

For many years, the practice had a flexible attitude to a catchment area. Many patients from the Ibrox and Govan areas had been rehoused in Castlemilk and Pollok, and they were given the option of remaining with the practice. Gradually, the time involved in house calls to Castlemilk and other outlying areas, such as Newton Mearns and Ralston, became hard to justify, as visits to these areas could involve a round trip of about an hour. A policy was established of requiring patients to move to a local practice if they changed address, even a change as minor as moving a few doors down the road and closer to the practice than other family members that had not moved. This proved to be extremely unpopular, and patients who remembered how Drs David Collins and Ockrim put patient loyalty above such considerations were deeply offended.

I phoned the doctor, and it was [because] my daughter was in another hoose. He turned roon' and said, 'Oh, you'll have to get off the surgery'. He never even gave her a prescription or a line for her work or nothing and away he went. . . . To me, it's no' [fair to have to] change your doctor. I've known you fae I was a wee lassie. It's a' right for him saying, oh you've flitted, you'll need tae change your doctor. That's no' the way tae deal wi' people. To me you're no' a doctor, tae me you're my friend as well as my doctor. . . . I could come in and talk to you. I told you all my problems.

(LD)

Glasgow GP and regular *BMJ* columnist Des Spence put the case for house calls very cogently and succinctly:[34] He argued that doctors were seeing patients only on 'our own consulting room turf, sanitised and controlled' and missing all the health care clues which came with a home assessment. In considering that 'the house visit is at the heart of medicine', he concluded that it forms an important and undervalued part of medical care.

Domiciliary Visits

In the early days of the British National Health Service, domiciliary visits were a continuation of the tradition, whereby general practitioners met consultants in the patient's home. This was sometimes seen as part of the GPs' education. One patient mentioned that a hospital consultant, a surgeon, had visited him at home, and the recommendation was that he should be admitted for further investigations. Consultants received a fee for the visit, and GPs generally valued the service whether or not they attended with the consultant. I have already referred to Frank Honigsbaum's paper on 'Quality in General Practice' which has a section on domiciliary consultations, a topic not covered in Loudon, Horder and Webster's otherwise very comprehensive coverage of general practice.[35]

Dr Collins, senior, came out to the house and said that he would like a surgeon from the hospital to come out and see me. Mr Tankel [the surgeon] came out to the house to see me. He said he would like me to come into the hospital so that he could examine me properly and do X-rays.

As the availability in general practice of hospital diagnostic services (radiology, bacteriology, pathology, haematology and biochemistry) increased, the need for a consultant visit to the patient's home declined except in very specific instances, usually related to geriatric medicine where the consultant sight of the patient's home could be relevant to the rehabilitation process.

These oral history testimonies showed the shape and content of general practice as seen by its consumers, the patients. These topics, open-access, appointments and organisational systems, all combined to contribute to the doctor–patient relationship. House calls have been and remain an essential component of family medicine, though the proportion of visits at home compared to consultations in the surgery continue to fall, with the now ubiquity of mobile phones and better patient mobility. The tensions over appointment systems and open access were finally resolved in the practice in favour of appointments but at a much later date than all other local practices. Patients valued their doctor's time and respected their opinions while looking on the surgery visit as a complete experience, which might include discussions in the waiting room and a nostalgic trip from a suburb back to the core of the practice area. We have also seen that it took many years for the role of a woman doctor in general practice to be routinely accepted.

NOTES

1 John Horder, Conclusion, in Irvine Loudon, John Horder, and Charles Webster, editors, *General Practice under the National Health Service 1948–1997* (Oxford University Press, Oxford, 1998), p. 282. Sarah Mitchell, Sarah Hillman, David Rapley, Sir Denis Pereira Gray, and Jeremy Dale, GP Home Visits: Essential Patient Care or Disposable Relic? *British Journal of General Practice*, 70 (695), 2020, pp. 306–307.

2 J. G. R. Howie, D. Heaney, and M. Maxwell, Quality, and Core Values and the General Practice Consultation: Issues of Definition, Measurement and Delivery, *Family Practice*, 21 (4), 2004, pp. 458–468; David Pendleton, Theo Schofield, Peter Tate, and Peter Havelock, *The New Consultation: Developing Doctor–Patient Communication* (Oxford University Press, Oxford, 2003).

3 *The Future General Practitioner: Learning and Teaching*, British Medical Journal [for] the Royal College of General Practitioners, 1972.

4 J. H. Levenstein, E. C. McCracken, I. R. McWhinney, M. A. Stewart, and J. B. Brown, The Patient-Centred Clinical Method: A Model for the Doctor-Patient Interaction in Family Medicine, *Family Practice*, 3 (1), 1986, pp. 24–30.

5 M. A. Stewart, What Is a Successful Doctor-Patient Interview? A Study of Interactions and Outcomes, *Social Science and Medicine*, 19 (2), 1984, pp. 167–175.

6 B. Guthrie and S. Wyke, Personal Continuity and Access in UK General Practice: A Qualitative Study of General 'Practitioners' and 'Patients' Perceptions of When and How They Matter, *BMC Family Practice*, 7, 2006, p. 11. https://doi.org/10.1186/1471-2296-7-11.

7 H. Hasegawa, D. Reilly, S. W. Mercer, and A. P. Bikker, Holism in Primary Care: The Views of Scotland's General Practitioners, *Primary Health Care Research and Development*, 6, 2005, pp. 246–254; Stewart W. Mercer, Peter G. Cawston, and Annemieke P. Bikker, Quality in General Practice Consultations; A Qualitative Study of the Views of Patients Living in an Area of High Socio-Economic Deprivation in Scotland, *BMC Family Practice*, 8, 2007, Article number: 22. https://bmcfampract.biomedcentral.com/articles/10.1186/1471-2296-8-22 (accessed 11 May 2020).

8 Anne Digby, *The Evolution of British General Practice 1850–1948* (Oxford University Press, Oxford, 1999), p. 199. She records that general practitioners were very accessible seven days a week. Saturday and Sunday evening surgeries were widely discarded after the World War II.

9 Anne Digby, General Practice 1850–1948, in *The Evolution of British General Practice*, p. 224.

10 Margery Spring Rice, *Working-Class Wives. Their Health and Conditions* (1st edition, 1939) (Virago, London, 1981).

11 Sara Arber and Lucianne Sawyer, Do Appointment Systems Work? *British Medical Journal*, 294, 1982, p. 480.

12 In the last days of the surgery in Cessnock Street in the winter of 1986/1987, water leakage from the vandalised roof caused patches of fungal growth on some of the ceilings and walls.

13 Jenny Field, Problems of Urgent Consultations within an Appointment System, *Journal of the Royal College of General Practitioners*, 30, 1980, pp. 173–177.

14 Henk Schers, Sophie Webster, Henk van den Hoogen, Anthony Avery, Richard Grol, and Wil van den Bosch, Continuity of Care in General Practice: A Survey of Patients' Views, *British Journal of General Practice*, 52 (479), 2002, pp. 459–462.

15 B. Guthrie, Does Continuity in General Practice Really Matter? Commentary: A Patient's Perspective of Continuity, *British Medical Journal*, 321, 2000, p. 734.

16 Shane W. Pascoe, Richard D. Neal, and Victoria L. Allgar, Open-access versus Bookable Appointment Systems: Survey of Patients Attending Appointments with General Practitioners, *British Journal of General Practice*, 54 (502), 2004, pp. 367–369.

17 D. C. Morrell, M. E. Evans, R. W. Morris, and M. O. Roland, The 'Five Minute' Consultation: Effect of Time Constraint on Clinical Content and Patient Satisfaction, *British Medical Journal (Clinical Research Edition)*, 292, 1986.

18 J. G. Howie, A. M. Porter, D. J. Heaney, and J. L. Hopton, Long to Short Consultation Ratio: A Proxy Measure of Quality of Care for General Practice, *British Journal of General Practice*, 41 (343), 1991, pp. 48–54.

19 Argyle Street: One of Glasgow's busiest shopping streets.

20 Fay Smith, Michael J. Goldacre, and Trevor W. Lambert, Adverse Effects on Health and Wellbeing on Working as a Doctor: Views of the UK Medical Graduates of 1974–1977: Surveyed in 2017, *Journal of the Royal Society of Medicine*, 110 (5), 2017, pp. 198–207. This survey of senior practitioners showed more stress in GPs than hospital doctors, with three-quarters reporting work stress and an imbalance between workload and home life.

21 When Dr David Collins retired, one of his patients recounted to me that his prescriptions were so good that 'we just put the prescription on the mantelpiece and when we looked at it, we always got better' (Personal recollection, 1978).

22 For an account of the doctor's gatekeeping role in certifying illness, see Anne Digby, *The Evolution of British General Practice*, pp. 252–254.
23 Nick Bosanquet and Chris Salisbury, The Practice, in Irvine Loudon, John Horder, and Charles Webster, editors, *General Practice under the National Health Service 1948–1997*, pp. 45–64. See also *Trends in General Practice* (Royal College of General Practitioners, London, 1977).
24 Morris McRae, *The National Health Service in Scotland: Origins and Ideals 1900–1950* (Tuckwell Press, East Linton, 2003), p. 228.
25 John Horder, Developments in Other Countries, in Irvine Loudon, John Horder, and Charles Webster, editors, *General Practice under the National Health Service 1948–1997*, pp. 271–272.
26 Nick Bosanquet and Chris Salisbury, The Practice, in Irvine Loudon, John Horder, and Charles Webster, editors, *General Practice under the National Health Service 1948–1997*, pp. 59–60; J. K. Hawley, I. S. L. Loudon, G. P. Greenhalgh, and G. T. Bungay, New Record Folder for Use in General Practice, *British Medical Journal*, (ii), 1971, pp. 667–670.
27 Nick Bosanquet and Chris Salisbury, The Practice, in Irvine Loudon, John Horder, and Charles Webster, editors, *General Practice under the National Health Service 1948–1997*, pp. 48–49, estimated the proportion at 25%, while a figure of nearer 33% was quoted in David Morrell's introductory chapter in the same book, p. 2.
28 See, for example, the NHS England GP contract. www.england.nhs.uk/gp/investment/gp-contract. The Scottish contract is framed the same way.
29 Sarah Mitchell, Sarah Hillman, David Rapley, Sir Denis Pereira Gray, and Jeremy Dale, GP Home Visits: Essential Patient Care or Disposable Relic? *British Journal of General Practice*, 70 (695), 2020, pp. 306–307. Also see J. Kaffash, GPs Vote for Home Visits to be Removed from Contract, *Pulse*, 22 November 2019. www.pulsetoday.co.uk/news/gps-vote-for-home-visits-to-be-removed-from-contract/20039743.article (accessed 31 March 2022).
30 Wikipedia. https://en.wikipedia.org/wiki/House_call (accessed 5 February 2020).
31 Ling Ling Soh and Lian Leng Low, Attitudes, Perceptions and Practice Patterns of Primary Care Practitioners towards House Calls, *Journal of Primary Health Care*, 10 (3), 2018, pp. 237–247. https://doi.org/10.1071/HC18022.
32 Ruth Abrams, Geoff Wong, Kamal R. Mahtani, Stephanie Tierney, Anne-Marie Boylan, Nia Roberts, and Sophie Park, Delegating Home Visits in General Practice: A Realist Review on the Impact on GP Workload and Patient Care, *British Journal of General Practice*, 70 (695), 2020, pp. 412–420.
33 M. F. Moore, J. H. Barber, E. T. Robinson, and T. R. Taylor, First-contact Decisions in General Practice: A Comparison between a Nurse and Three General Practitioners, *Lancet*, 301 (7807), 1973, pp. 817–819.
34 Des Spence, Doctor in the House, *British Medical Journal*, 346, 2013, p. 1809.
35 F. Honigsbaum, Quality in General Practice. A Commentary on the Quality of Care Provided by General Practitioners, *Journal of the Royal College of General Practitioners*, 22 (120), 1972, p. 437.

5

Stigma and Marginalisation

The NHS's building programme created an infrastructure which eventually ended the relationship between certain hospitals and the old poor law institutions, but new forms of stigmatising behaviour emerged. As we shall see, the sense of shame associated with stigma could still be felt many decades later. While one might expect that families and friends might rally round the stigmatised individual, they might also be the very people who have borne the brunt of the negative behaviours associated with alcohol or drugs.

Despite the Scottish sense of openness, represented by 'we are all Jock Tamson's bairns', there is a long history of incoming groups feeling isolated from the mainstream, being different due to religion, race or language.[1] To understand how stigma functioned in the experience of the participants in the study, we must first see how the topic is defined and then understood in the extensive academic literature.[2] The data is interpreted and displayed in a clinical manner.

DEFINITIONS OF STIGMA AND MARGINALISATION

In an article on stigma and social identity in 1963, Goffman described 'stigma' as an interactive social process whereby an individual is deeply discredited by society because of a perceived personal attribute or behaviour, creating a 'spoiled identity' imbued with social failing.[3] Almost forty years later, Link and Phelan indicated that social science research on stigma had grown dramatically in the past two decades. They define 'stigma' as occurring when labelling, stereotyping, separation, status loss and discrimination are present, and indicate that for stigmatisation to occur, power must be exercised.[4] Stigma, therefore, calls into question a person's moral character, behavioural choices and their right to full membership in society. Such people can then be devalued or rejected.

The testimonies show, for example, the relationship of tuberculosis and schizophrenia to stigma, while many other illnesses are free of that association. Finally, say Link and Phelan, there can be no stigmatisation without the fifth component of stigma, the exercise of power.[5] As stigma can be used to control, exploit or exclude others, people may have an interest in using stigma power to put people down or away. Link and Phelan claim that stigma is frequently the power mechanism of choice and may even be used covertly. Finally, they show that because there are so

DOI: 10.1201/9781003369301-5

many stigmatised circumstances, stigmatisation can have a dramatic bearing on all the aspects of life chances, both social and health.

Feelings of stigma can influence behaviour, create anxiety, reduce interaction with other people and compromise recovery prospects. Many social stigmas are embedded in popular culture and may relate to gender and race as well as health.[6] Therefore, Link and colleagues note, difficulties faced by stigmatised individuals clearly define stigma as a society rather than an individual problem.[7]

In the interviews, we encounter memories of means-tested benefits, social welfare provision of inferior housing, and paternalistic and parsimonious provision of children's clothing and other items remain fresh. Some stigmas are related to health, tuberculosis, psychiatric illnesses and physical deformities; and some to behaviour which falls outside society norms, like addiction and homosexuality; and finally, some to being a member of a group, nationality, religion or race which is seen as 'different'.[8]

Stigma Themes

The data obtained from the oral history study will show what stigma means to the participants and how it was experienced. The lessons learned from the testimonies will show how this study adds to other research on the topic. In the interviews, the effects of stigma stretch beyond the individual, and often, the main locus of the stigma is felt within the family. Victorians tended to divide the poor into categories of deserving and undeserving, the latter being especially disadvantaged. The interviews show that though the experience of being stigmatised may affect self-esteem, academic achievement and other outcomes, I will show how many people who experienced stigma have retained high self-esteem, showed resilience to their negative experiences and often managed to have high attainments at work and in the wider society.

Though the era and attitudes of the past which produced the attribution of stigma may have disappeared, the hurt still remains part of an individual's emotions and beliefs. Consequently, health care organisations have developed strategies for supporting clients that feel their views or their worth are not being properly respected.[9] There is already some sign that campaigns, such as the See Me project in Scotland and the Glasgow Anti-Stigma Partnership, which bring these issues into the open in a positive way, is having some effect.[10]

This study shows that it took some time before the sense of stigma disappeared from the Glasgow hospitals which had been involved with Poor Law health care.[11] The poor were not required to be housed in poorhouses, as in England, but could be given relief in cash or kind.[12] The Scottish poorhouses were intended for the sick and destitute poor, and catered extensively to those suffering from mental illness, and provided very basic accommodation with asylum and infirmary beds.[13] The Govan Combination Poorhouse (later the Southern General Hospital) served the parishes of both Govan and Gorbals. The poorhouses were intended for the sick and destitute poor, and inmates of these poorhouses were segregated into male and female areas, and this segregation continued into differentiating between the deserving and non-deserving poor. These buildings catered extensively to those suffering from mental illness and provided very basic accommodation, though with asylum and infirmary beds.[14]

One participant (BC) recalled the effect on her family of being placed in the Foresthall Home and Hospital[15] due to temporary homelessness caused by a flood in their home. Foresthall had a fearsome reputation, while it operated as a poorhouse, for the harsh conditions in which the inmates were forced to live and work.[16] She recalled how she and her children had been made homeless by a major storm in 1968 which severely damaged their building. BC described the primitive conditions and the behaviour of long-term residents as 'an eye opener', indicating that this was a highly inappropriate housing placement.

We have descriptions of the numerous former mental asylums in the Greater Glasgow area and can try to understand what life was like for individuals living in these fearsome institutions.[17] Participants reported that the stigma that they or their families felt about mental illness was related to what was experienced in prison-like conditions, often far from home. Many of the great Victorian asylums had extensive grounds, and Climie described the way that, even today, property developers who are trying to sell houses on the land of former mental institutions are coy about mentioning the real history of these sites. The old asylums around Glasgow, Gartnavel, Woodilee and Hawkhead claimed to offer a quiet and peaceful environment and a self-supportive community lifestyle to aid recovery. Nevertheless, all were associated with stigma.

POVERTY STIGMA

Several participants described how they had felt a poverty stigma from the way in which they were treated by the authorities and by how they saw themselves regarded in their local society. One woman, brought up in a single-parent home, following the death of her father just weeks before her birth, recalled the extreme poverty of the 1930s. At the same time, this testimony shows how the welfare provided was also stigmatising. GR explained how her mother relied on the 'Parish' and 'had to sell all her furniture' and had to 'use orange boxes instead'. While there was food poverty at home, it was the clothing that was stigmatising. She recalled the embarrassment of welfare clothes because 'Everyone knew that was the sign of parish clothes—poverty, and I mean poverty'.

The assessment of entitlement to benefit by the means test was also felt too demeaning. Rules were applied strictly and often in an unfeeling way. JR struggled to help her brother-in-law financially, but the means test inspector's response was 'if you can't keep him on that we can put him in to Foresthall'.

INSTITUTIONAL STIGMA

The local hospital, the Southern General, had begun as a poorhouse, while the Victoria Infirmary, to the east of the practice area, had been a private hospital, supported by patient charges as well as charitable donations. Admission there did not have the same stigma attached to it. Participants were quite clear that there was a stigma attached to the Southern General—'that this was still a place that wasn't supposed to be talked about'.

> It was always the Victoria he recommended. You see, my father was very much against the Southern General. He said to my mother, 'Don't put me in the poorhouse.' It had this sort of stigma to it. It all changed, but the older people thought that this was still a place that wasn't supposed to be spoken about.
>
> (RM)

> The only thing I remember is, my father talking about the Southern General—a Parish Hospital and he wisnae keen on going in.
>
> (JC)

There was also a hierarchy of clinics for outpatient treatment in the pre-NHS days. The Victoria Infirmary had a dispensary in the practice area—'at the bowling green in Bellahouston Park'—while nearby, in Summerton Road, was the parish clinic which was associated with the poorhouse, marginalisation and stigma. As FN recalled, 'The very bottom used to be the poorhouse [clinic]'.

ILLNESS STIGMA

Tuberculosis

Tuberculosis was the illness most frequently cited in the oral histories as the classic stigmatic disease. It was especially common in Glasgow. The decades before, the National Health Service had seen disappointing figures for the prevalence of tuberculosis in Glasgow, though mortality levels had been falling, but there were better results for the other infectious diseases, such as measles and whooping cough.[18] However, it was the association of tuberculosis with so many of Glasgow's social and health ills that made it a special case and was more associated with stigma. Tuberculosis, as the commonest cause of death in young adults, was rightly feared in Glasgow.

Jacqueline Jenkinson devoted a lengthy chapter on tuberculosis, its management and consequences, in her *Scotland's Health 1919–1948* (Peter Lang, Bern, 2002). She notes that it took the reform of National Insurance in 1946 to provide disability benefits for all TB patients and that in 1948, almost a tenth of all deaths in Glasgow were due to tuberculosis.[19] As senior medical students in the early 1970s, we were not even allowed to mention the word 'tuberculosis' in a patient's hearing, referring to the condition as Koch's disease, after the pathologist Robert Koch, who identified the tuberculosis bacillus. The disease was rife in the city, and the sense of stigma was its association with overcrowding in tenement homes and, in the pre-chemotherapy era, memories of morbidity and mortality in sufferers. By 1951, more than half of all cases of TB in Scotland could be found in Glasgow and surrounding burghs. Neil McFarlane has argued that it was not poor nutrition which was the major factor behind Glasgow's resurgent TB in the 1930s and 1940s but rather the small, crowded tenement houses.[20] Lilli Stein convincingly showed, in 1952, that respiratory TB incidence and mortality rates were highly correlated with both overcrowded homes but less so with poverty and unemployment.[21]

It was believed that rest and fresh air, which were provided in Glasgow at Ruchill, Mearnskirk and Philipshill Hospitals, could assist the healing process. The facilities at Mearnskirk were impressive and included a surgical unit for treatment of tuberculosis complications. McFarlane noted that, with the opening of the facilities at Mearnskirk in 1932, Glasgow had the best level of TB bed provision in the country and yet was unable to improve treatment outcomes. In patients with a positive finding of the TB bacillus in the spit, for the years 1935–1938, almost three-quarters were dead within five years.[22] McFarlane concluded that it was cheaper to hospitalise patients than deal with the underlying social problems.[23]

In the pre-antibiotic era, treatment for TB could mean years in an institution, often with lengthy and painful treatment for its lengthy complications if the patient survived. As the 1950s progressed, TB became a treatable condition managed at the outpatient chest clinic. The first drugs for TB were frequently described as wonder drugs: streptomycin and PAS (para-aminosalicylic acid), from 1945, when combined with streptomycin, was found to greatly reduce the occurrence of drug resistance. In 1952, isoniazid (INH) became available. The three drugs were often prescribed together.

The family and personal experience of tuberculosis had a pervasive effect on many of the interviewees, and the length of time confined to sanatorium or hospital had major effects on subsequent lives, and the stigma of the disease could not be ignored. The stigma operated at two levels. Firstly, there was the association of TB with inferior and overcrowded housing with conditions which increased the risks of transmission and reinforced societal attitudes against patients. Secondly, there was the self-image of patients with the disease who had allowed the diagnosis to affect their sense of worth, producing shame and fear.[24]

In this testimony, ZI recalls that 'nobody spoke about it' and that it was 'a taboo subject'. He remembered that his mother refused accommodation to a young family member with TB through fear of transmission:

TB was the stigmatic thing. Nobody spoke about it. I knew plenty people who had TB, thankfully nobody in my family. TB was a taboo subject because a family who had a person with TB, and sometimes there's more than one, they didn't want to know because then they would be known as an unhealthy family and another family wouldn't want to be married into, which was quite ridiculous. Oh, there was a member of my family who had it—a cousin from Edinburgh. Again, this was something I found quite hurtful at the time. Nobody would have him: he died because nobody really cared enough.

The sense of stigma was pervasive. BE recalled that 'if you heard that somebody had TB, you used to think that was terrible', while GD acknowledged that 'there was always fear of infection in the house', and 'there was an unclean sort of feeling about it. It was a terrible disease, and they had no answer to it at that time'. ISo said that she was so concerned about the stigma of TB that when she went on the tramcar to the clinic, 'I went past the stop because I didnae want him [the driver] to see where I was going. Just because it was TB'. Patients were aware that TB patients were not being given the diagnosis. RNr remembered that when she 'was a young girl, tuberculosis was a bad word. Consumption they called it. That was a bad word'.

IT had all the investigations and treatment associated with TB without the stigmatising word 'tuberculosis' being mentioned, although by this time, the name 'streptomycin' was synonymous with the disease. Even when TB could be cured by medication, the stigma persisted, and HS was only told that 'they discovered it . . . just like two tiny pieces of thread just over the top of both lungs'. EL admitted that she had hardly known any close family with TB because 'I'm going back to pre-war, and you weren't told about things'.

LNd said she was told that she had 'hip-joint disease because I don't think anyone mentioned the word tuberculosis in those days'. She felt marginalised by the city's Education Department who refused her admission to Bellahouston Academy, where the science class was in a different building. Despite pleading that she was fit enough to walk from one building to the next, the head teacher suggested that her father 'just put her into some domestic thing where she can learn to sew and cook'. Attitudes gradually changed with the introduction of chemotherapy, and GR was made to feel privileged that she could be treated with treatment at her local hospital rather than be transferred to the sanatorium environment at Mearnskirk.

Tuberculosis still destroyed families in the first half of the twentieth century. Patients who were diagnosed with tuberculosis by the 1960s were often picked up by a programme of routine X-rays. In 1957, an intensive five-week campaign was launched in Glasgow to identify TB carriers in the city.[25] Thirty-seven mobile radiography units, manned by volunteers, visited housing schemes, offices and factories with the initial aim of X-raying 250,000 people. However, intense media coverage, support of community activists and a weekly prize draw from the names of those who came forward helped raise the number of screenings to nearly 715,000. Confirming this, GT said that her TB was 'brought to light by the mass x-rays. It was done at work'.

Rickets

In the years after World War I, there was an ongoing medical controversy about the cause of rickets. Dietary factors seemed to be important, but it was not until 1973 that it was understood that proper exposure to sunlight was required to produce the vitamin D that was necessary to prevent rickets. Rickets was a common scourge of children in the Glasgow tenements where sunlight was extremely limited.[26] As we will see, the condition began to be diagnosed more recently with significant numbers of patients from the Indian subcontinent, unused to the Scottish weather, settling in the area.

In earlier times, the association of rickets with slum dwellers and poor diets meant that the condition carried a social stigma so that parents often sought an alternative diagnosis, like bow-leggedness.[27] Bow-leggedness (*genu varum*) is a deformity marked by outward bowing at the knee causing the lower leg to be angled inwards. In Glasgow, the main cause of the condition was rickets, but infants can have a degree of bow-leggedness which disappears as steady walking is established. One mother came to Dr Ockrim, worried about the stigma associated with rickets:

[My son] had legs like barrels. The Green Lady told me it was rickets, and I went along to you, and I said, 'The Green Lady said he had rickets.'. . . You said, 'Let him walk'. I told him to walk. You said, 'Rickets! what is she talkin' aboot? She doesnae know what she's talkin' aboot. He's no' got rickets. He's bow-legged, but he doesn't have rickets.'

(JB)

Concealed/Denied Pregnancy

One significant carrier of stigma until the last decades of the twentieth century was the unmarried mother. Society has now come to acknowledge the mental trauma caused to women who had children out of wedlock. These testimonies speak of the time when having a child outside marriage was deeply stigmatising for the whole family. They describe the solutions which families sought—to have the baby born out of Glasgow, to arrange adoption or, if the baby was to remain within the family, to be brought up as the youngest child of the baby's grandmother. Though there was often some sympathy for wronged women, too often, they were seen as sinners that had earned community disapproval.

Fear of stigma could lead to a concealed pregnancy where a woman who knows that she is pregnant does not tell any health professional. She may confide that she is pregnant to another person but still not access any antenatal care or make contact with any health agencies. A denied pregnancy is where a woman is either unaware that she is pregnant or is unable to accept the existence of her pregnancy. There may be health or psychological reasons for either of these situations, and there is an extensive literature on the topic, much of it from health agencies concerned about the risks to mother and child.[28] IN described the situation of only finding that her daughter was pregnant when Dr Ockrim examined her and said, 'Yes, she is pregnant and she's in labour. She's havin' a baby'. I said, 'Dear God!'

ZT described herself as a 'gullible' youngster, unaware that she could be pregnant, saying that 'I had never had intercourse'. Her father had to be told not to chastise her, and what happened to her was as follows:

was put into the Tor [Christian] Nursing Home in Edinburgh. That was six months pregnant right up until the baby was born and it got adopted.

Other families could be more pragmatic. IK was determined to stand by her pregnant unmarried daughter and had resigned herself to the baby being adopted out of the family. However, at the last minute, the daughter decided not to go through with the adoption, and the baby was brought up in IK's home, and 'He gets the attention and love that all kids need'.

MENTAL HEALTH, ADDICTIONS AND STIGMA

Mental health occupied a somewhat peripheral place in medicine in the first decades of the twentieth century. Significant psychotic episodes had to be treated with custodial care, and psychiatric hospitals, formerly known as lunatic asylums, had a fearsome reputation. Memories of mental illness in the family could cast a long shadow.

> There's a few tragedies. Granny had a young son who had a nervous breakdown . . . and Granny was trying to cover up. It was Leverndale and she didnae want anybody to know. I think he was only a young boy when that happened. It was months and months. I think it was a stigma on some people. That must have been part of Granny's generation. Anything else can be wrong with them as long as it's no' a mental illness.
>
> (IK)

One of the participants had been a male nurse in the Hawkhead Asylum in the 1930s, when the extensive hospital grounds contained a farm with over a hundred cattle. In the days before the State Hospital at Carstairs opened to cater for the criminally insane, Hawkhead dealt with inmates on murder charges. One of the participants had been a male nurse at Hawkhead (DS), and he described the conditions which produced the stigma associated with these asylums. He recalled strict regimes for patients and staff, and remembered patients coming from Barlinnie Prison in straightjackets. At this point, Dr Ockrim recalled that during her undergraduate psychiatric training, she was at Hawkhead, and she thought the practice of displaying the patients to see them perform foolish actions was degrading and very cruel. She remembered as follows:

> some of them used to do silly things and the nurses or doctors would ask them to do things and they would do things, and everybody laughed as if it was a joke.

DS agreed, saying that in the lecture room, the following happened:

> they would maybe have the epileptics in, and they would maybe have ten of them in and he would have them all doing this and that with their ear. One fellow could flap his ear, and this caused a laugh of course.

Schizophrenia

Many schizophrenics are devalued and discriminated against because of their mental illness. Dickerson and colleagues reported that patients may have heard offensive statements and media accounts about their condition, noting that socio-economic variables, but not symptoms or social functioning measures, were related to the extent of stigma and discrimination experiences.[29] Ertugrul and Uluğ related society stigma to those with more severe symptoms, such as depression and active social avoidance. This relationship between the perception of stigma and symptoms of disease is a vicious circle in which the elements reinforce each other and hamper recovery.[30]

This next extract is the voice of a parent (ZN) who feels he has to navigate a Kafkaesque world in understanding his son's schizophrenia and providing a safe home environment for him. He was clear about the stigmatising nature of the illness and pointed to examples from his contact with the Schizophrenic Fellowship, the family support group:

> The time I have to try and change some of the things you see. The big problem as I see it is not schizophrenia in my mind, it's attitudes. We have as an organisation a tremendous potential. We cannot get people to come out into the open. We have people who come to us for help, but they don't want us to send them anything. They don't want anyone to know.

The patient's father recalls the history of his son's illness and relates how he involved himself with family support groups and also read widely in detailed psychiatric texts. It is an important account of the development of a complex mental illness with its frequent relapses into unpredictable behaviour with all the aspects which engender stigmatisation. When his son was arrested, in the 1960s, during an episode of euphoria, the court showed little understanding at first till he gave evidence:

> I explained to them, a bit about schizophrenia . . . and they listened very patiently. It was very good. The main factor was that there was a lot of ladies in the court. I could feel the sympathy as I talked and the magistrate said, 'Well, I understand the situation very well now.' He said: 'I'm not going to fine you because I know you are an ill young man, but this is the third time you've been here and if you come back again there's just nothing I or anyone else can do, you'll end up in prison.' He said, 'So I see no sense in giving you any punishment whatever, go with your father and listen to him.'

The story also shows the patient's struggles with his parents, and especially his father, to come to terms with it and the encounters with both general practitioner and hospital services. The insightful commentary of the father and his sometimes cynical views of the professionals engaging with his son, both in the practice and in the hospital, give the narrative an enduring quality of how paranoid illness affects the wider family. Yet the family never give up on their disturbed son who is marginalised by his illness and lives in a solitary state that few can understand.

> We went in to see the psychiatrist and his attitude was hostile to me—not with me. . . .
> Well, there's hardly a panel in our house which wasn't fractured. . . . His obsession was the media, which is not uncommon. The television interfered with his thoughts. All forms of media was a threat to him. His concentration went away as far as reading was concerned. Televisions got smashed. I think we had three smashed. He was tremendously guilty afterwards.

All my collection [of books] which never done me much good was all gathered one night, quietly and all burned. The psychology books, psychiatry books. They were all taken out and burnt. That didn't bother me too much.

My view now of schizophrenia is that I'm a part of my son's illness, my wife's a part of my son's illness, his friends and relatives are part of it, his GP's a part of it and his psychiatrist is a part of it and it's the way we respond to his illness is for good or better.

(ZN)

Depression

Depression has also come to be seen as stigmatising, mostly in relation to employment and access to health services but additionally within the family circle.[31] The economic cost of depression and its impact on society have prompted studies on how stigma can be reduced. One recent Scottish study indicated how methods to measure the economic impact of anti-stigma campaigns are scarce and proposed a model for testing.[32] One patient described how people might have thought she had been 'in the loony bin'. Two patients described the unsympathetic attitude of their employers, and one, the unfeeling attitude of a hospital nurse, while the final memory showed the limits of sympathy to a real mental health illness within the family.

I went back to work [after about] nine months and. . . . I had to get my courage back to face my workers and my neighbours. I thought at that time, 'It's silly, I know—[but they might be thinking] Oh she's been in the loony bin'. I thought that people wouldnae understand that there was nothing wrong and I was just exhausted.

(FS)

The next memories describe the sense of shame associated with depression and the unfeeling attitudes of those in authority which compounds the problem. Depressed patients found it impossible to admit to a stigmatising illness which was affecting the standard of their work. GD admitted this:

Everything seemed to be getting on top of me. . . . Maintenance which I believed should have been done was being pushed aside and I used my own men and trained them to do the necessary preventative maintenance and I was stopped doing that.

RN described how she had experienced 'a terrible depression' while working as a home help. Her supervisor 'wasn't terribly sympathetic and she would say, 'You'll just have to cope, it's as simple as that''. But RN said, 'I got to the stage I couldn't cope. What I would have to do in two hours, I was trying to fit into an hour'. She needed time off work and a course of antidepressants to recover.

ZR described the details of his wife's depression which began after a mastectomy, treated with lithium and ECT. He recalled this:

If she had died in her sleep, I would have been relieved. I knew she couldnae go on the way she was going. . . . When this started, I went to drink and then she died. I was drinking a bottle of whisky a day. Prior to that they had told her that they didnae think it was any relation to this breast off. They felt that it was building up in her. It may have triggered her off, but it wasn't the cause of it. She was going to have this sort of breakdown anyway.

While these three experiences of depression do not mention the word 'stigma', the idea was very much in the participants' minds.

Dementia

Dementia is now a major cause of disability in the elderly, and Milne, who has written extensively on wellbeing in mental health, described it as 'one of the most serious challenges facing the older population, their families and health and social care services in the developed world'.[33] Dementia has been declared a national policy priority and that 'reducing the high levels of stigma' associated with the condition is one of the key objectives of the National Dementia Strategy. Swaffer has described how dementia affects a person's willingness to seek diagnosis, to seek support once diagnosed and to participate in research. She also notes that the care provided is of a lower standard due to stigma within the health care professions. Services become distorted, and she quotes studies which show how stigma increases the feelings of shame, both towards the patient and by the patients themselves. Indeed, writing from personal experience of stigma and discrimination since acquiring the various disabilities of dementia, she points out that it is the carer's voice which remains dominant in dementia and stigma literature.

In 1990, more than 1% of Scotland's population had dementia, and by 2020, the proportion was approaching 2%, mostly resulting from Alzheimer's disease. It may take some time before a diagnosis of dementia can be made with confidence, and there has been debate on the appropriate time for patient and family to recognise that the condition is present.[34] Early diagnosis can reduce uncertainty about accepting the diagnosis, exclude rare but treatable causes, provide patient and family support, and help to avoid crises. Diagnosis can also create anxiety and depression, and for some, this carries a stigma.

Studies in Scotland have also confirmed that general practitioners have a central role to play in the effective primary care response to people with dementia and their families, while noting the concern about the adequacy with which they fulfil this role.[35] At the Midlock Medical Centre, we took a pro-active role in the identification and management of its patients with dementia. In addition, I was employed by the Dementia Services Development Centre at the University of Stirling to bring good dementia practices to general practitioners around Scotland since GPs perceive considerable difficulties with some aspects of dementia care, and accordingly, they require a range of interventions that would assist them.[36]

The following memories show the feelings of guilt experienced by carers and the difficulties in providing an acceptable level of care at home and even making sure that the patient remains safe as her memory deteriorates. We see the struggle of daughters to provide care and the feelings of guilt and shame as they realise that their mother has to enter a residential home. Then there is the son who works out of town and has difficulties in helping his mother cope with declining mental function.

I remember one night she started. By this time, she was in a bed with the sides drawn up. Oh yes, she was becoming demented. . . . It wasn't her. . . . The doctor called one day and took a look at me and said, 'We've got to do something.' I still feel terribly guilty.

(LG)

She [my mother] had taken a slight stroke on the Monday and on the Tuesday, she took a massive one and she was put into the Southern General. . . . From there, they tried to rehabilitate her back home again, but she was too badly disabled. Because of my circumstances, she actually died in Crookston Home. . . . [It was] awful. I couldn't visit her. I would go in and I would run out the door, because I was so guilty. . . . But it's just when I get talking about it, I think, 'How could I have done that?'

(EX)

From it started—I saw the signs about five months before it started. . . . Mother was always close to me, and I wondered what was wrong and then I realised that something was happening within her own brain that was causing this. I leave sufficient food in the house [when I'm away] but there are times when I come back up, the food's not been touched, so there are days she's not eating.

(QD)

Addiction

Loudon, Horder and Webster's book on *General Practice under the National Health Service 1948–1997* has no reference to drug addiction, alcoholism or cigarette smoking in its index. These following testimonies, full of raw emotion, indicate that addictions are a key element of general practice care and that stigma is a major factor in its various forms. There are many recollections of difficult, almost impossible, times in dysfunctional families, relieved only by the story of those who managed to cure their addiction. This might be through family admonition, Alcoholics Anonymous or, in the case of cigarettes, enlightened self-interest. The doctor's role has been to listen, understand, counsel and support and, at the same time, realise that the patient might go straight from a warning about problem drinking to the nearest pub.

Addictions are commonly accompanied by a sense of shame or self-stigmatisation. This results from public attitudes which lead the addict to internalise the negative stereotype that society associates with addiction.[37] Thus, public opinion in stigmatising and marginalising the addict, whether due to alcohol or drugs, feeds into the addict's reduced sense of self-worth. Hay and colleagues at the Glasgow Centre for Drug Abuse noted that labelling people as 'problems' meant that they were seen as separate from mainstream society.[38]

In some cases, patients found relief with self-help groups, such as Alcoholics Anonymous. However, it was often the resulting damage to families, from violence, separation and financial loss which were the predominant memories.

Alcoholism

The World Health Organisation defines 'alcoholics' as follows:

> those excessive drinkers whose dependence on alcohol has attained such a degree that they show a noticeable mental disturbance or an interference with their bodily and mental health, their personal relations and their smooth social and economic functioning, or who show the prodromal signs of such a development. They therefore need treatment.[39]

Acceptance by the patient of the label 'alcoholic' has been viewed by many practitioners as a prerequisite to alcohol abuse recovery. However, the label is seen as a highly stigmatised term associated with people that have lost homes, livelihoods and family due to alcohol. An Editorial in the *British Journal of Addiction* in 1987 considered that 'the term 'alcoholism' . . . has now been largely discarded' as a word 'synonymous with the disease of alcoholism'. The word 'alcoholic' has become a term of abuse symbolising the problem drinker, while most people in Britain accept that drinking alcohol has an important social function. This was underlined by the Royal College of Psychiatrists, who removed the term 'alcoholism' from the second edition of their policy statement on alcohol in 1986:

> There are good reasons for calling into question the continued usefulness of a word which is all things to all men, laden with mythology, and sometimes cruelly unkind to the person [through] stigmatisation.[40]

There were many examples of the behaviour of alcoholic patients which demonstrate how the habit came to be associated with stigma in families, at work and in society. These memories describe the problems related to excess alcohol consumption and explain why the associated behaviours are stigmatising. VF said that he was drinking 'every waking moment'. He did not want to:

> get taken into hospital, so I pooh poohed it until such times as a bed had to be found for me. . . . I woke up in Leverndale one morning. I was pretty bad. It was an institution—a psychiatric pit. There was a reception area of all the nervous disorder people, court cases, alcoholics and general inadequates of society.

VF found that he could turn his life round and move forward free of the stigma that his excessive drinking had provoked by attendance at Alcoholics Anonymous (AA), and at the time of the interview, he had been sober for thirty-one years. He remarked, 'I'm not confident, just vigilant against the first drink'.

ZT admitted that she never sees her brother:

because he turned out to be a complete rogue. He's never out the jail and I just don't want that type of person. My father put him out when he was seventeen. He was stealing [from] my father. And he was breaking into houses. I kept him for a year and then put him out. He was stealing and lying.

HN mentioned a father who recovered through working with down-and-outs at the Salvation Army, and LD described the problems related to her marriage to a binge drinker.

It was maybe every three months; he would take a drink and when he went out with his friends, he would take a drink maybe every three months or even six months. He wouldnae hit you but he would throw things about, and I just gave him an ultimatum. I said, the next time you dae that, I'm no' goin' oot the house, you can please yourself. You either stop going oot wi' your pals and stop drinkin' or I don't come back wi' the kids. Ever since that he's never touched a drink.

Drug Addiction

Drug addiction in the Govan area increased substantially during the 1970s and 1980s. Many lives were blighted, and some addicts died young as a result of complications with intravenous injections or from overdoses of the abused drugs. Suddenly, doctors in the practice were assailed by young patients looking for addictive prescription drugs, such as benzodiazepines and dihydrocodeine. These could be abused or sold to fuel the habit of illicit drugs.[41] Studies confirmed the extent of drug abuse in Glasgow, noting both that deaths occurred in a younger age group compared to other cities and that mortality rates among drug abusers were higher.[42] By late teens or early twenties, problems of drug abuse and criminality will be well established and difficult to rectify.

Nordil suggested that the origins of the stigmatisation of council housing tenancies followed the large-scale slum clearances, the movement to large-scale housing estates and the failure of central and local government to recognise the signs of social breakdown.[43] One of the areas in Govan mentioned by participants was the Moorpark estate but better known as Wine Alley, where alcoholism and drug addiction became rife and often associated with the social conditions that it represented, producing both stigma and marginalisation of the residents. Situated just a mile west from Midlock Street, it was considered Britain's most notorious housing scheme.[44] Drug-related crime was common, and police would only enter in twos with another car on standby. A damning indictment of officialdom was contained in a report by Sean Damer, a social scientist who spent six months living there in 1975.[45] With no communication between planners and residents, fundamental errors in managing the properties were constantly perpetuated. Eventually, the placement of social misfits, who could not be housed elsewhere, destroyed the area, and it was demolished in the late 1990s. Today, the area houses some small business workshops.

There was an awareness that the problem called for drastic solutions, and the response in Glasgow was the formation of the Glasgow Drug Problem Service

(GDPS) in 1994, just a couple of years after the oral history project concluded.[46] The Service organised the use of oral methadone to enable many opiate dependent drug injectors to reduce or cease injecting, with the hope of improvements in health and social stability. The scheme was widely adopted, as it was seen as a huge improvement on the previously chaotic state in Glasgow, but there was also widespread scepticism about the efficacy of methadone substitution and reservations about its benefit remain. Drug-related deaths in Scotland have been increasing sharply, numbering 1,330 in 2021, having increased more than five-fold since 1996. This was more than three times the level in England and Wales, and very much the worst in Europe. Around a third of these had lived in the Greater Glasgow and Clyde Health Board area, which has less than a quarter of Scotland's population.

The practice had many patients in Wine Alley, and for the most part, they differed little from the patients in the neighbouring areas. However, as increasing numbers of people with social problems were given housing there, older patients were very aware of the addicts in their midst.

> You hear of some of the young ones in the scheme. You hear about them mostly up at Wine Alley. I think that's where a lot of it goes on. . . . I suppose there's a lot of decent folk up there too. It's just the same everywhere.
>
> (BE)

> There's a drug addict [in the building]. She doesnae affect me. I'll talk to them. They don't bother with me. I don't bother. She's been there for about eleven years. She was in with the jags and that. You know when she's high. There's quite a few of them. That's the Wine Alley over there. Well, they're emptying half of that I hear. . . . It's Moorpark now. There are nice people over there. I've met quite a lot and I think they are nice.
>
> (ISo)

It took some time for the practice to create coping mechanisms for dealing with the drug addicts and their behaviours. Policies had to be established for finding out who was entitled to be seen as a patient. Because of the abuses of the system, including lying and forging prescriptions, such patients were frequently removed from GP lists. As drug addicts found major problems in registering with a different practice, they would be allocated to a named practice, usually for a period of three months. Unfortunately, it often took three months for case notes to reach the new practice, and the receptionists had to obtain the necessary accurate information before the doctor could see the patient. Sometimes false information was given which would lead to a fruitless search for accurate information.

> At the beginning I never really noticed the drug addicts but now we get more and more. They get put off one list, so they've got to be put on to some doctor, so we find we get quite a lot of them. You try and keep as calm as you can. Most of the time they are not [abusive], and they are demanding to be seen then and there. You try and explain things to them and keep your patience with them.
>
> (Joan Kilcullen, Receptionist)

You are very aware of the problem [of drug addiction] here. You see so many—we get at least three or four a week. It's quite frightening sometimes because you don't know how they are going to react to you. If they are told they have not to join the list for some reason, they can become quite violent. They refuse to leave the surgery and on a lot of occasions we've had to call the police in. You've got to learn to deal with it. Drunks are different, you can sort of humour them, and they tend to just go away.

(Sandra Grant, Receptionist)

Well, we have quite a lot of problems with prescriptions from addicts—whether they are taking the drugs themselves or selling the drugs on the street, we're not terribly sure. The policy of the Practice now is that when a new patient or a temporary resident patient comes and the girls are suspicious of them, we have a typed note to say that as a Practice we do not prescribe certain drugs. These drugs are named, and these are the drugs that the drug addicts want. This in a way helps but if it's our own patients, we find that all the drug addicts around here know each other and if the surgery doesn't have a strong policy as regards withholding certain drugs, then they would all actually come to this surgery or come to whatever surgery they found easiest to get drugs. We have had patients apprehended from the surgery, but this has been known patients to the surgery who have come in and we knew that they were actually wanted by the police.

(Nanette Aitken, Practice Manager)

Receptionists would check with Health Board records to confirm the addict's story, only to find that the name of the doctor given was fictitious or that, commonly, there was no record of registration with a practice. The addict would then be informed that they would need to contact the Health Board themselves and that they would then be allocated to a practice.

We've got about a dozen [drug addicts] or thereabouts. . . . The doctors tend to keep them under control. The doctor gives us the prescription, we take it round to the chemist, the chemist them gives the patient the tablets. It is in case they are actually altering the prescription itself.

One patient was issued a prescription and went to the local chemist and before she had time to get it dispensed, when she was still in the shop, we realised that she shouldn't have had the prescription because of her history. . . . So, I rushed round to the local chemist and took the prescription out her hand, and she was left standing without it.

(Nanette Aitken, Practice Manager)

Patients began to report that their children, other close family members or neighbours had become addicts. Their constant need for money to buy illicit drugs led to petty criminality, often shoplifting but frequently, too, selling off prized possessions within the home.

If my daughter was in the house . . . we were so silly taking her back. Learn to be harder hearted. Having to lift your purse when you go to the toilet. It's horrible when you can't trust who's living in the house with you. I can't describe it to you. It makes a cloud in the house and the atmosphere. You're listening to her saying something and you think to yourself, 'Is that the truth or is it a lie?' You can't believe anything they say and you've to watch what they're going to do.

I couldn't talk about it at all. It was horrible. You felt ashamed. I was blaming myself that she went to the drugs and all that and yet I know in my heart. . . . When I used to go up [to the surgery], I'd be sitting there and I'd say, 'Oh God, there's one of my daughter's pals'. You could spot a junkie a mile off. I just hated being in the same room as them. It was a horrible feeling, you know.

(LB)

Yes, I've came across it because one of my sons was on it and ended up getting septicaemia and had to get new valves in his heart . . . the doctor [said] 'It's septicaemia he's got and he hasnae got very long'. . . . It was a Prof, and he came and spoke to me in the hospital. He said, 'You know, this treatment costs an awful lot of money, and do you think that he'll have learned his lesson, if we put all this work and effort in to making him better'? I said, 'I think he looks as if he's learned his lesson'.

(IN)

The boy above me died through one of them. He injected himself. He used to come to my door. In fact, he set his room on fire the night he came here. He used to come here—Well you know the drugs my husband was on. He was on morphine, DF's as they call them.[47] . . . This boy used to say, 'I'll gi' ye' a pound for a tablet'. . . . I wouldn't give them a tablet. I gave him [a] cigarette and he went away up and went to sleep on his drugs and set the bed on fire. . . . The place was in flames. I was lucky I never got injured.

(LN)

Quite a few in the street have died wi' drugs. You see them coming up in the cars and there's a boy who used to be across there who lifted the windae a wee bit—selling them out the windae.

The police didn't seem to be interested. They would come but they seemed to know when the police were coming. . . . There was a shooting a fortnight ago, through drugs. Shootin' from flats to a guy in a car. You've no idea what it's like there.

(LI)

Drug addicts also came into contact with the medical services through faulty injection techniques which resulted in abscesses and other complications. Often, these had to be dealt with by the district nurse:

The drug people—abscesses on their arms, legs, thighs. We wear gloves for all dressings now. We are told we must use gloves for all dressings. We would also wear an apron and have the special disposal bags for contaminated waste to make sure that it is properly disposed of. . . . One boy I remember—he seemed very pleasant to talk to, but he had a massive, big abscess and he was living with his girlfriend and two young children in the house. The house was—there was nothing in it.

(Sister Mary Cowan)

When asked if she would report such things to the Social Work Department, Sister Cowan replied as follows:

No. The problem is if we were going about doing these things, we would probably not get back into the home again. You have got to be careful. It's difficult. Unless they actually ask for some help—then you would refer them to a social worker.

The final recollections come from patients that had seen drug dealers and users in their neighbourhoods. These include comments about their perception of inadequate police responses.

Well, there is a problem. There is drugs gettin' sold aboot here. You see the needles everywhere. You see them gathering in wee groups and the fancy cars coming. We don't know who they are. They're all strangers. [The police come] occasionally, but they're no' around a great deal. It's all stopped recently in this area. I don't know what's happened. It's all calmed doon in this particular bit. I seen them [the addicts] stoatin' aboot and I seen the needles lyin' aboot, but I've never had any bother wi' them.
  I phoned the police once because there was a really bad fight at the corner. . . . The next morning, I went oot all the boys were shoutin', 'Oh there's a grass in that close.' It's no' right. . . . The only time the police bother is if there's a murder getting done. . . . It's a waste of time.

(LD)

If you are in the pub, you hear all kinds of things. Thae shopping centres and different places—there's certain ones [drug pushers] hanging about there all the time. I often wonder [why the police can't spot them]. . . . The pubs in Nitshill—it was a well-known fact that every pub had them. The police must know that. At times I think they do [turn a blind eye]. That's my opinion.

(ID)

These memories of the problems of drug addiction mostly refer to the behaviours which stigmatise the abusers of illegal substances. Solutions proved to be beyond the scope of individual practices who sometimes were overwhelmed by the demands posed by addicts. At the same time, regular users of the medical services clearly saw all these behaviours as stigmatising.

Cigarette Smoking

In Robert Proctor's book *Golden Holocaust: Origins of the Cigarette Catastrophe and the Case for Abolition*, the cigarette is described as the 'deadliest artifact in the history of human civilisation'. The dangers of cigarette smoking had been identified in

Germany in the 1930s, but it was not until 1950 that papers began to appear in the British and American medical journals warning about smoking and lung cancer.[48] Positive associations were found for various cancers, chronic obstructive pulmonary disease and other respiratory diseases; for vascular diseases and, perhaps because of confounding, by personality and alcohol use, from cirrhosis, suicide and poisoning. Stopping smoking before middle age could eliminate almost all the risks, and even some reduction could confer partial benefit. Doll and colleagues estimated that about half of all regular cigarette smokers would eventually be killed by the habit.

Toleration to nicotine may occur, and withdrawal symptoms can last for some time and can be quite troublesome. There may also be some additional behaviour factors in the addiction.[49] Because of the awareness of the health risks of cigarette smoking and its increasing social unacceptability, there has been a significant decline in the number of smokers. At the same time, it is becoming recognised that cigarette control strategies have led to a situation where the smoking has become stigmatised, especially among the disadvantaged groups where the habit mainly persists.[50]

Cigarette smoking had been recognised as the single most important contributor to ill-health in Scotland, with economic costs to the smoker and society, and increased demands on health care resources.[51] While primary health care team professionals in Scotland were strongly committed to health promotion and smoking cessation, constraints of time and lack of training proved barriers to success. Opportunistic health promotion, of which smoking cessation is a major part, was recommended as a regular part of the work of practice nurses, health visitors and general practitioners, while Health Boards were setting up their own clinics which allowed a better engagement with patients.

> I said, I'm not going to smoke any more but after four weeks of boredom and missing my cigarettes, I lit up and my husband was absolutely flaming mad . . . he stopped twenty or thirty years ago. Every time I took a cigarette he would say, 'Yes, you go on smoking, it'll help you nicely'. I had plenty of warning and I didn't listen. . . . I really feel young people in school should be warned how dangerous. . . . How you did this for years and not think you would do any damage.
>
> (DT)

> What I didn't like [in the hospital] was . . . everyone from all around about came into that ward and smoked. You could cut the atmosphere with a knife in it. I had just stopped smoking and I found it most annoying—the amount of smoke. I kept opening the window and arguing with people in the ward. They were shouting to shut the window. . . . The rule was that they were supposed to smoke after meals, but they smoked from—all day.
>
> They spoke to this man next to me about smoking in bed. I was concerned because there was oxygen there. . . . In fact, him and I had words about it. Slightly more than words. I had him round the throat. I was gonnae throw him out the window. I threatened to throw him out the window and then I calmed down.
>
> (HT)

Robert Proctor observed that no other industry had shown such disregard for the welfare of its customers. Recent years have seen more decisive action to curb smoking, through restrictions on advertising and sports sponsorship, and crucially, a ban on smoking in pubs and restaurants. These measures, with the health promotional activities in GP surgeries and special clinics have all had some impact on the prevalence of cigarette smoking. As the numbers of cigarette smokers have declined in recent years, studies have indicated that the social stigma faced by cigarette smokers, as smoking is removed from public venues, has sharply increased. Hilary Graham described the decline in cigarette smoking in high-income countries, attributed to 'the increasing social unacceptability of smoking, a cultural shift in which tobacco control policies are identified as playing a major part'.[52]

Studies have already shown that smoking stigma may prevent smokers from consulting a physician and induce alternative tobacco product use to aid cessation.[53] Public health authorities have stressed the need to counteract stigma in order to promote better public health. At the same time, stigma is being employed as part of society's attempts to push cigarette smoking beyond the barrier of normal behaviour.[54] However, this view has been challenged by Bell and colleagues who felt that stigmatising smokers would not reduce smoking prevalence in the disadvantaged groups that represent the majority of smokers. They considered that it might actually limit access to health care efforts in primary care.[55]

Marginalisation

The large immigration from the Indian subcontinent produced an increasingly ethnically diverse population in the practice which requires cultural sensitivity.[56] The practice learned how to meet the challenges of dealing with immigrant health issues, often related to conditions such as heart disease, diabetes, tuberculosis and rickets, and requiring reduction of any stigma associated with immigration. However, Glasgow had attracted other immigrant groups, such as the Irish, Italians and Eastern European Jews who had also experienced discrimination, stigmatisation and marginalisation.[57]

Some of the patterns of illness in the South Asian population differed from that found in the other practice patients.[58] Over the years, various attempts were made to try and tackle health inequalities in this population group, concentrating on such illnesses as cardiovascular disease, hypertension and diabetes mellitus. A few patients arrived with symptoms of tuberculosis. It had also been known for some time that Asian Indians who immigrate to Northern Europe have lower serum vitamin D than Caucasians, and they are thus prone to develop vitamin D deficiency, rickets and osteomalacia. Further studies established the extent of the problem in Glasgow.[59] Within a few years, the addition of vitamin D supplements had eliminated the prevalence of florid rickets in the Asian children.[60] The Glasgow campaign showed that even suboptimal vitamin D supplementation greatly reduced the prevalence of severe rickets in Asian children, and it was extended to Asian women who continued to show evidence of vitamin D deficiency leading to osteomalacia.[61]

The interviews showed how the theme of marginalisation was felt by patients whose ethnic or religious background placed them outside what they perceived to be the mainstream. One of the Jewish interviewees felt marginalised because of his background which held a different attitude to social drinking.

> When I worked with the Scottish Radio Orchestra, at lunch time we would go out and have six pints and then come back and play and play well. They are heavy drinkers. When I first went into television drama, the head of television drama invited me for lunch and a drink. I said, 'I don't drink at lunch time.' He said, 'I don't trust people who don't drink.' There is that attitude in our society that drinking is part and parcel of our social life—especially in areas where it is very attention filled. In the acting, writing, music world—it's so fraught with uncertainty that people do drink and do drugs.
>
> (ZT)

In the next memory, we see how Dr Ockrim's own religious identity was questioned by a patient's priest. However, she was fully supported by the patient who would not allow the priest to marginalise the views of her doctor.

> I remember this time that the priest had come in and he was talking to me about the children. Me having had four sections, I was worried about children, and I happened to say to the priest about having children. I said to him that my doctor was worried, and I was not to have any more children. He said to me, 'What religion is your doctor?' I said, 'The doctor is a Jew.' He said, 'Oh, you should get yourself a Catholic doctor.' I said, 'What difference does that make?' He said, 'Oh, the Catholic doctors will understand you better.' I said, 'I wouldn't swap my Jewish doctor for anything.' He said, 'He doesnae understand.' I said, 'Well my Jewish doctor is better than any of your Catholic doctors.'
>
> (BC)

From a medical point of view in the practice, the majority of the Protestant population and the minority Catholic community had similar views and outlooks, although we will see some issues relating to Protestants giving birth at the St Francis Nursing Home.

A German woman, who had married a Scot at the end of the war and settled in Glasgow, said the following:

> I wasn't made very welcome by my in-laws. My mother-in-law . . . just about tolerated me because I was married to her son.
>
> (DT)

The increasing numbers of mainly Pakistani Muslims in the Govan area, with their different skin colour, language, religion, dress and customs, created a big impact on the neighbourhood.[62] By the time the interviews were being conducted, patients of South Asian origin made up around 12% of the practice numbers, reflecting almost exactly their proportion in the local population. Though serious racial incidents were reported to be few, or mainly of a minor nature, violent episodes did occur. Qualitative data collected specifically in Edinburgh suggest that Muslims visibility has triggered some ethno-religious discrimination.[63]

A local pharmacist, who was interviewed as a patient in the practice, noted this:

There was a definite ethnic change. There was a lot of Asians came into the area. It brought us in a lot more prescriptions. I think they made good use of the health service. I am not saying they didn't need it, but they certainly used it.

(IS)

A few patients mentioned the presence of Asian patients in the waiting room talking in their native languages. Dr Ockrim was sensitive to the question of racial prejudice and took issue with one the interviewees.

The only incidents I see is when the Paki's are in, and they are talking in their own language. I did see one of the receptionists telling them to keep to English when they're in there. That was the only time.

>Dr: *But the thing is, some of them can't speak English.*
>I never thought of that.
>Dr: *Do you think they may be saying something against you?*
>I think it gives you an inferiority complex, as if they're speaking about you.
>Dr: *So how would you feel now about listening to them speaking their own language?*
>I don't suppose it would bother me now that it's been pointed out to me.
>Dr: *So, do you think a lot of the racial feeling is that people don't understand and don't know and there should be a lot more understanding?*
>Yes, I do.
>Dr: *Have you ever heard some of the girls [in the office] speaking Gaelic in the surgery?*
>No.
>Dr: *Well they do. So how would you feel about that—Do you think you would feel the same way about that?*

The only fault [in the surgery] is, when you are sitting in there, these Asian patients—When they are all speaking it's like a constant drone. I mean they're pleasant. I would never ignore them. I speak to them and that if they've spoken to me.

(RNr)

The only thing I didn't like was in the old surgery—The Asians used to come in and there used to be two in front of you and another two would come in and another two—six or eight of them would walk into the room at once. . . . The Asians you couldnae talk to. They just wernae interested in having a conversation. There's only one Asian person I've ever met, and she was a chatty person and that was round at the bus stop. She was saying, 'Where do you live?—That's a nice scheme'. We chatted away.

(LG)

I get on with them ok. Here and there they will call me black B's and this and that, but that's only to make me angry more than anything else—to get their anger out of them and trying to make me angry. Jealous—yes. People are jealous for a lot of different reasons. They maybe think—right—I'm standing in the shop and the till is going ding-ding, ding-ding—I'm making a lot of money and the person in the street is unemployed. He can't make any money— He can't get any job. I'm to blame for that. Well, I'm not to blame for that. He doesn't know that I'm there from six o'clock in the morning till six o'clock at night. I know that all I'm getting at the end of the day is wages.

No, I don't think [there's a racial problem] in Glasgow. Definately not.[64] I've had my problems—I've been mugged in my shop. They steal from me. I wouldn't say that was due to racial.

(LB)

I was working the buses and I never seen anything. If they did, I don't mind because in Pakistan, there is good and bad people all over the place, so I don't notice.

(LC)

One time a boy in another class hit him with a bottle on the head. I went to the headmaster. The headmaster was very good. They told me not to worry about it. He knows all the family. He called the police, and the police took action.

(LC)

A younger Asian participant (FC) who had experience working as a social worker had her own view on the racial prejudices she had encountered, which included people saying, 'You should go back to your own country'. She and her husband made the decision to send their children to private schools where she felt that though there was still an element of racial prejudice, 'if we've left our own country, we want our kids to be brought up with good manners'. Alcohol in society was seen as a problem:

When we do visit them, alcohol is involved in it. We feel that we are left out at a function and it's not the right place for us to be, but we do go up with a gift and come back very early. . . . [I have] been to functions where they are drunk.

(FC)

Abstention from alcohol was so ingrained in the local Muslim community that when a patient of the practice developed alcohol-related cirrhosis of the liver, there was some disbelief at first, and while the family provided exemplary care as their relative died from complications of liver failure, it was obvious that the family felt a stigma. Some of the men might have a drink away from home, but an illness related to prolonged heavy, and necessarily secret, drinking was hard to cope with.

The story of a teenager exemplified a lot of these issues, and her father (LB) was keen to portray his opinion on the matter, as her behaviour related to stigma within his family and community and reflected the interaction of immigrant parents and the next generation. The practice, as the story unfolds, tried to maintain close touch with parents and daughter, providing valuable support and understanding for father and daughter.

> They were sent to the mosque when they were young. They read the *Koran*—they all have their own books. I request of them that once or twice a week they should read their books. They done it in their own time. I didn't say, 'Look sit down and read.' It was put into their mind that if they read it is good for them. [She] was always quite a nice girl and she had a very good report from the school. Always happy, and the teacher was always very pleased with her.
>
> Very helpful at home. Good at school. Never said no to her mother, never said no to anybody in the class. Apparently, there was a girl in that school who we had heard from people that she was not good to be friendly with. . . . We never had any problem with [her], but slowly and slowly that girl got working on [her] and she was sort of misleading [her]. Then all of a sudden, one morning [her younger brother] came from the school and told me she was not in the class,

When her parents disciplined her, the situation spiralled out of control. Her father admitted that his wife had 'hit her a couple of times' and said that, if truanting did not stop, he would 'break every bone in [her] body'. The school nurse, the head teacher and social workers were all involved, though following a review by the police, the court reporter and the social worker, no further police action was taken. However, to the parents' surprise but with his daughter's agreement, the social worker arranged admission to a children's home. The family was much more accepting of the situation when she continued to show her attachment to her faith. The home gave her a self-catering room and allowed her weekly access to the mosque.

> I spoke to her about her marriage, and I told her—In fact I went back and told my mother and father as well. Nearly all my relations know now. My mother and father know, and they said, 'Look when the time comes for her marriage—If she can get married to a Muslim child, she will get together again.' That is their judgement. I would agree with that, and I think that is the only hope . . . if she would get married to someone non-Muslim then I'm afraid I don't want to see [her] at all.
>
> (LB)

All the patients quoted in this chapter saw themselves as part of the mix that makes up Scottish society, sometimes described as threads in the tartan. As first-generation immigrants, the participants of Pakistani origin saw many things in their background and beliefs that they wished to maintain. In this they saw themselves as marginal to the mainstream of Scottish society with which they wished to integrate. At the same time, they had to acknowledge that pressures from the society outside would mean the making of some compromises while struggling to keep red lines in place. Stefano Bonino argues that it is hard to gauge the extent of anti-Muslim sentiment in Scotland and that the goal should be the reduction of discrimination where it occurs while maintaining Muslim distinctiveness within Scottish society.[65]

Stigma continues to exist as a society response to a range of diseases and behaviours. Various strategies have been suggested to deal with this. These include improving knowledge about the issues through the media, having campaigns like See Me, having training programmes and removing barriers, legal and employment, which reinforce stigma. These testimonies show how stigma and marginalisation impacted on the lives of the study participants. It requires work with stigmatised individuals to engender a feeling of self-worth and personal responsibility, and a greater awareness in society about reducing stigmatising attitudes.

NOTES

1 See my *Be Well! Jewish Immigrant Health and Welfare in Glasgow 1860–1914* (Tuckwell Press, East Linton, 2001), especially: Jews and Hospitals, pp. 91–92; Trachoma in Glasgow 106–111; Mental Health, pp. 115–130; Jews and the Medical Missions, pp. 155–172.

2 *Chronic Ill-Health*: Valerie A. Earnshaw, Diane M. Quinn, The Impact of Stigma in Healthcare on People Living with Chronic Illnesses, *Journal of Health Psychology*, 17 (2), 2011, pp. 157–168; Neville Millen and Christine Walker, Overcoming the Stigma of Chronic Illness: Strategies for Normalisation of a 'Spoiled Identity', *Health Sociology Review*, 10 (2), 2014, pp. 37–40; Ann Jacoby, Dee Snape, and Gus A. Baker, Epilepsy and Social Identity: The Stigma of a Chronic Neurological Disorder, *Lancet Neurology*, 4 (1), 2005, pp. 171–178; Kelly L. Andrews, Sandra C. Jones, and Judy Mullan, Stigma: Still an Important Issue for Adults with Asthma, *Journal of Asthma and Allergy Educators*, 4 (4), 2013, pp. 165–171.
Mental Health and Addiction: Peter Byrne, Psychiatric Stigma: Past, Passing and to Come, *Journal of the Royal Society of Medicine*, 90, 1997, pp. 618–621; S. Clement, M. Jarrett, and C. Henderson, Messages to Use in Population-Level Campaigns to Reduce Mental Health-Related Stigma: Consensus Development Study, *Epidemiology and Social Psychology*, 19 (1), 2010, pp. 72–79; L. Knifton, M. Gervais, K. Newbigging, and N. Mirza, Community Conversation: Addressing Mental Health Stigma with Ethnic Minority Communities, *Social Psychiatry and Psychiatric Epidemiology*, 45, 2010, pp. 497–504; I. McPhee, A. Brown, and C. Martin, Stigma and Perceptions of Recovery in Scotland: A Qualitative Study of Injecting Drug Users Attending Methadone Treatment, *Drugs and Alcohol Today*, 13 (4), 2013, pp. 244–257.
Tuberculosis: L. Mtui and W. Spence, An Exploration of NHS Staff Views on Tuberculosis Service Delivery in Scottish NHS Boards, *Journal of Infection Prevention*, 15 (1), 2014, pp. 24–30; J. Macq, A. Solis, and G. Martinez, Assessing the Stigma of Tuberculosis, *Psychology, Health and Medicine*, 11 (3), 2006, pp. 346–352; Patricia Kelly, Isolation and Stigma: The Experience of Patients with Active Tuberculosis, *Journal of Community Health Nursing*, 16 (4), 1999, pp. 233–241; Susan Kelly, Stigma and Silence: Oral Histories of Tuberculosis, *Oral History*, 39 (1), 2011, pp. 65–76.
Other Illnesses: Elinor Devlin, Susan MacAskill, and Martine Stead, 'We're Still the Same People': Developing a Mass Media Campaign to Raise Awareness and Challenge the Stigma of Dementia, *Journal of Philanthropy and Marketing*, 12 (1), 2006, pp. 47–58; Stigma and Misconceptions Are Critical Barriers

to Reach HIV Targets in Scotland, 2018, *International Association of Providers of AIDS Care*, www.iapac.org/2018/10/29/stigma-and-misconceptions-are-critical-barriers-to-reach-hiv-targets-in-scotland/; Roy G. Beran (Editorial), Discussing the Risks Related to Epilepsy—An Holistic Approach, *Seizure: The European Journal of Epilepsy*, 2020, pp. 134–135. https://doi.org/10.1016/j.seizure.2020.02.04.

Poverty Stigma: G. Inglis, F. McHardy, E. Sosu, and J. McAteer, Health Inequality Implications from a Qualitative Study of Experiences of Poverty Stigma in Scotland, *Social Science and Medicine*, 232, 2019, pp. 43–49; B. Watts, Rights, Needs and Stigma: A Comparison of Homelessness Policy in Scotland and Ireland, *European Journal of Homelessness*, 2013, p. 48, ISSN 2030–2762/ISSN 2030–3106 online.

Marginalisation: N. Quinn, Participatory Action Research with Asylum Seekers and Refugees Experiencing Stigma and Discrimination: The Experience from Scotland, *Disability and Society*, 2014; S. Bonino, Scottish Muslims through a Decade of Change: Wounded by the Stigma, Healed by Islam, Rescued by Scotland, *Scottish Affairs*, 24 (1), 2015. www.euppublishing.com/doi/abs/10.3366/scot.2015.0054 (accessed 27 March 2022); L. Knifton, Understanding and Addressing the Stigma of Mental Illness with Ethnic Minority Communities, *Health Sociology Review*, 21 (3), 2014, pp. 287–298; P. C. Gronholm, C. Henderson, and T. Deb, Interventions to Reduce Discrimination and Stigma: The State of the Art, *Social Psychiatry and Psychiatric Epidemiology*, 52, 2017, pp. 249–258; R. Davidson, Psychiatry and Homosexuality in Mid-Twentieth-Century Edinburgh: The View from Jordanburn Nerve Hospital, *History of Psychiatry*, 20 (4), 2009, pp. 403–424.

3 Erwin Goffman, Stigma and Social Identity, in Tammy L. Anderson, editor, *Understanding Deviance: Connecting Classical and Contemporary Perspectives* (Routledge, New York and London, 2013), p. 256ff.

4 Bruce G. Link and Jo C. Phelan, Conceptualizing Stigma, *Annual Review of Sociology*, 27, 2001, pp. 363–385; B. G. Link and J. C. Phelan, Conceptualising Stigma, *Annual Review of Sociology*, 27, 2001, pp. 363–385; L. H. Yang, A. Kleinman, B. G. Link, J. C. Phelan, S. Lee, and B. Good, Culture and Stigma: Adding Moral Experience to Stigma Theory, *Social Science and Medicine*, 64 (7), 2007, pp. 1524–1535.

5 B. G. Link and J. Phelan, Stigma Power, *Social Science and Medicine*, 103, 2014, pp. 24–32.

6 Cathy Campbell and Harriet Deacon, Unravelling the Contexts of Stigma: From Internalisation to Resistance to Change, *Journal of Community and Applied Social Psychology*, 16 (6), 2006, pp. 411–417.

7 Bruce G. Link, Jerrold Mirotznik, and Francis T. Cullen, The Effectiveness of Stigma Coping Orientations: Can Negative Consequences of Mental Illness Labeling Be Avoided? *Journal of Health and Social Behavior*, 32 (3), 1991, pp. 302–320.

8 Cathy Campbell and Harriet Deacon, Unravelling the Contexts of Stigma: From Internalisation to Resistance to Change, *Journal of Community and Applied Social Psychology*, 16 (6), 2006, pp. 411–417.

9 The Scottish Association for Mental Health (SAMH) maintains a website titled See Me which shows what stigma might look like and gives examples of how clients might be affected by unfeeling attitudes and indicates good practice. Issues included their concerns being dismissed by professionals, being treated as a diagnosis rather than a person, not being listened to,

having false assumptions, being fobbed off with medication, being dismissed as attention seeking. Access at www.seemescotland.org/health-social-care/information-for-people-using-health-and-social-care/experiencing-stigma-and-discrimination-in-health-and-social-care/.

10 See Me; 2011. Access at: www.seemescotland.org; N. Mehta, L. Kassam, G. Butler, and G. Thornicroft, Public Attitudes towards People with Mental Illness in England and Scotland, 1994–2003, *British Journal of Psychiatry*, 194 (3), 2009, pp. 278–284; 9. L. Dunion and L. Gordon, Tackling the Attitude Problem. The Achievements to Date of Scotland's 'See Me' Anti-stigma Campaign, *Mental Health Today*, 40, 2005, pp. 22–25. See also Neil Quinn and Lee Knifton, Glasgow Anti-Stigma Partnership: A Five-year Programme Report. https://pureportal.strath.ac.uk/en/publications/glasgow-anti-stigma-partnership-a-5-year-programme-report (accessed 27 March 2022).

11 See Clifford Williamson, 'To Remove the Stigma of the Poor Law': The 'Comprehensive' Ideal and Patient Access to the Municipal Hospital Service in the City of Glasgow, 1918–1939, *History: The Journal of the History Association*, 99 (334), 2014, pp. 73–99.

12 David Hamilton, *The Healers: A History of Medicine in Scotland* (Canongate, Edinburgh, 1981), pp. 229–233.

13 Ibid.

14 Ibid.

15 Formerly the Barnhill Poorhouse. In 1945, it was renamed Foresthall Home and Hospital. It remained under the control of Glasgow Corporation after the NHS began.

16 *The Workhouse in Barony, Glasgow*: www.workhouses.org.uk/Barony/ (accessed 14 February 2021).

17 Paul Climie, Asylums in Glasgow: The Buildings Where Madness Was Managed. https://sourcenews.scot/asylums-in-glasgow-the-buildings-where-madness-was-managed/ (accessed 31 May 2021); https://canmore.org.uk/site/44226/glasgow-1345-govan-road-southern-general-hospital (accessed 23 January 2019).

18 Cristopher Clayton, Tuberculosis, in Gordon McLachlan, editor, *Improving the Common Weal: Aspects of Scottish Health Services 1900–1984* (Edinburgh University Press, Edinburgh, 1987), pp. 383–410.

19 Jacqueline Jenkinson, *Scotland's Health 1919–1948* (Peter Lang, Bern, 2002), pp. 327–329.

20 Neil McFarlane, Hospitals, Housing, and Tuberculosis in Glasgow, 1911–51, *Social History of Medicine*, 2 (1), 1989, pp. 59–85.

21 L. Stein, Tuberculosis and the 'Social Complex' in Glasgow, *British Journal of Social Medicine*, 6, 1952, pp. 1–48.

22 Report of the Scottish Health Services' Council's Committee on Tuberculosis (Edinburgh, 1951), Appendix 14a, p. 60.

23 Neil McFarlane, Hospitals, Housing, and Tuberculosis in Glasgow, p. 85.

24 *TB Stigma Measurement Guidance*. www.challengetb.org (accessed 22 October 2020).

25 www.nhsggc.org.uk/about-us/history-of-the-nhs-in-greater-glasgow-and-clyde/70th-anniversary-of-the-nhs/70-years-of-the-nhs-in-greater-glasgow-and-clyde/1948-1950s/1948-1950s/1957-chest-x-ray-campaign-helps-to-eliminate-tb-in-glasgow/# (accessed 22 March 2021).

26 Morrice McCrae, *The National Health Service in Scotland: Origins and Ideals: 1900–1950* (Tuckwell Press, East Linton, 2003), pp. 48–49, 144. McCrae

quotes levels of 70% in some Central Scotland districts. Helen Dingwall, David Hamilton, Iain Macintyre, Morrice McCrae and David Wright describe in *Scottish Medicine: An Illustrated History* (Birlinn, Edinburgh, 2011), that rickets 'was a major cause of sickness and deformity among children' from the last half of the nineteenth century.

27 In the various accounts of the history of medicine in Scotland, only Helen Dingwall and Morrice McCrae mention rickets as a public health issue: Helen Dingwall, *A History of Scottish Medicine: Themes and Influences* (Edinburgh University Press, Edinburgh, 2003), p. 167 and Helen Dingwall et al., *Scottish Medicine*.

28 See, for example, Susan Hatters Friedman, Amy Heneghan, and Miriam Rosenthal, Characteristics of Women Who Deny or Conceal Pregnancy, *Psychosomatics*, 48 (2), 2007, pp. 117–122.

29 Faith B. Dickerson, Jewel Sommerville, Andrea E. Origoni, Norman B. Ringel, and Frederick Parente, Experiences of Stigma among Outpatients with Schizophrenia, *Schizophrenia Bulletin*, 28 (1), 2002, pp. 143–155.

30 Aygun Ertugrul and Berna Uluğ, Perception of Stigma among Patients with Schizophrenia, *Social Psychiatry and Psychiatric Epidemiology*, 39, 2004, pp. 73–77.

31 Carol Roeloffs, Cathy Sherbourne, Jürgen Unützer, Arlene Fink, Lingqi Tang, and Kenneth B. Wells, Stigma and Depression among Primary Care Patients, *General Hospital Psychiatry*, 25 (5), 2003, pp. 311–315.

32 P. McCrone, M. Knapp, M. Henri, and D. McDaid, The Economic Impact of Initiatives to Reduce Stigma: Demonstration of a Modelling Approach, *Epidemiologia Sociale*, 19 (2), 2010, pp. 131–139.

33 Alison Milne, The 'D' Word: Reflections on the Relationship Between Stigma, Discrimination and Dementia, Editorial, *Journal of Mental Health*, 19 (3), 2010, pp. 227–233.

34 Steve Iliffe, Jill Manthorpe, and Alison Eden, Sooner or Later? Issues in the Early Diagnosis of Dementia in General Practice: A Qualitative Study, *Family Practice*, 20 (4), 2003, pp. 376–381.

35 M. Downs, The Role of General Practice and the Primary Care Team in Dementia Diagnosis and Management, *International Journal of Geriatric Psychiatry*, 11, 1996, pp. 937–942; M. Downs, I. Cook, C. Rae, and K. E. Collins, Caring for Patients with Dementia: The GP Perspective, *Aging and Mental Health*, 4, 2000, pp. 301–304. Midlock Medical Centre took a pro-active role in the identification and management of its patients with dementia. Case finding through the home-visiting screening by a practice nurse led into initiatives for management.

36 M. Downs, A. Cook, C. Rae, and K. E. Collins, Caring for Patients with Dementia: The GP Perspective, *Aging and Mental Health*, 4 (4), 2000, pp. 301–304.

37 S. Matthews, R. Dwyer, and A. Snoek, Stigma and Self-Stigma in Addiction, *Bioethical Inquiry*, 14, 2017, pp. 275–286.

38 G. Hay, M. Gannon, N. McKeganey, S. Hutchinson, and D. Goldberg, *Estimating the National and Local Prevalence of Problem Drug Misuse in Scotland* (Centre for Drug Misuse Research, Glasgow 2005). www.drugmisuse.isdscotland.org/publications/local/prevreport2004.pdf.

39 A. B. Sclare, The Epidemiology of Alcoholism, *British Journal on Alcohol and Alcoholism*, 13 (2), 1978, pp. 86–92. (Quoting the World Health Organisation, Expert Committee on Mental Health, Alcoholism Subcommittee, Second Report, 1952, Geneva. Techn. Rep. Serv. 48.)

40 Editorial, No 'Alcoholism' Please We're British, *British Journal of Addiction*, 82, 1987, pp. 1059–1060.

41 Richard Hammersley, Alasdair Forsyth, and Tara Lavelle, The Criminality of New Drug Users in Glasgow, *British Journal of Addiction*, 85 (12), 1990, pp. 1583–1594.

42 Martin Frischer, David Goldberg, Mohammed Rahman, and Lee Berney, Mortality and Survival among a Cohort of Drug Injectors in Glasgow, 1982–1994, *Addiction*, 92 (4), 1997, pp. 373–506.

43 E. Nordil, *The Origins of the Double Stigma of Large Post-War Council Estates in the UK: 1945–1978*, 2018 Master's Thesis, University of Oslo, duo. uio.no (accessed 27 March 2022).

44 http://citystrolls.com/life-in-wine-aley/wine-alley-revisited/ (accessed 3 June 2019).

45 Sean Damer, *From Moorepark to 'Wine Alley': The Rise and Fall of a Glasgow Housing Scheme* (Edinburgh University Press, Edinburgh, 1989).

46 Laurence Gruer, Philip Wilson, Robert Scott, Lawrence Elliott, Jayne Macleod, Kenneth Harden, Ewing Forrester, Stewart Hinshelwood, Howard McNulty, and Paul Silk, General Practitioner Centred Scheme for Treatment of Opiate Dependent Drug Injectors in Glasgow, *British Medical Journal*, 314, 1997, p. 1730; P. Wilson, R. Watson, and G. E. Ralston, Methadone Maintenance in General Practice: Patients, Workload, and Outcomes, *British Medical Journal*, 309, 1994, p. 641.

47 DF118: Dihydrocodeine tartrate, indicated for severe pain and popular with opioid addicts.

48 R. Doll and A. B. Hill, Smoking and Carcinoma of the Lung. Preliminary Report. *British Medical Journal*, ii, 1950, pp. 739–748; E. L. Wynder and E. A. Graham, Tobacco Smoking as a Possible Etiologic Factor in Bronchogenic Carcinoma, *Journal of the American Medical Association*, 143, 1950, pp. 329–336; R. Doll and A. B. Hill, The Mortality of Doctors in Relation to Their Smoking Habits. A Preliminary Report, *British Medical Journal*, i, 1954, pp. 1451–1455; R. Doll, R. Peto, K. Wheatley, R. Gray, and I. Sutherland, Mortality in Relation to Smoking: 40 'Years' Observations on Male British Doctors, *British Medical Journal*, 309, 1994, p. 901.

49 Faraz Mughal, Smoking Reduction during Ramadan, *British Journal of General Practice*, 67 (659), 2017, p. 254. Suriani Ismail, Hejar Rahman, Emelia Zainal Abidin, et al., The Effect of Faith-Based Smoking Cessation Intervention During Ramadan among Malay Smokers, *Qatar Medical Journal*, 2016 (2), 2016, p. 16; Reuven Dar, Florencia Stronquin, Roni Marouani, Meir Krupsky, and Hanan Frenk, Craving to Smoke in Orthodox Jewish Smokers Who Abstain on the Sabbath: A Comparison to a Baseline and a Forced Abstinence Workday, *Psychopharmacology*, 183 (3), 2005, pp. 294–299.

50 M. Graham, Smoking, Stigma and Social Class, *Journal of Social Policy*, 41 (1), 2012, pp. 83–99.

51 A. Scott Lennox and Ross Taylor, Smoking Cessation Activity within Primary Health Care in Scotland: Present Constraints and Their Implications, *Health Education Journal*, 54, 1995, pp. 48–60.

52 Hilary Graham, Smoking, Stigma and Social Class, *Journal of Social Policy*, 1 (1), 2012, pp. 83–99.

53 Brown-Johnson, G. Cati, and Lucy Popova, Exploring Smoking Stigma, Alternative Tobacco Product Use, and Quit Attempts, *Health Behavior and Policy Review*, 3 (1), 2016, pp. 13–20.

54 Ronald Bayer, Stigma and the Ethics of Public Health: Not Can We But Should We, *Social Science and Medicine*, 67, 2008, pp. 463–472.

55 Kirsten Bell, Amy Salmon, Michele Bowers, Jennifer Bell, and Lucy McCullough, Smoking, Stigma and Tobacco 'Denormalization': Further Reflections on the Use of Stigma as a Public Health Tool. A Commentary on *Social Science & Medicine*'s Stigma, Prejudice, Discrimination and Health Special Issue (67: 3), *Social Science & Medicine*, 70 (6), 2010, pp. 795–799.

56 Raj S. Bhopal, The Quest for Culturally Sensitive Health-Care Systems in Scotland: Insights for a Multi-Ethnic Europe, *Journal of Public Health*, 34 (1), 2012, pp. 5–11.

57 Kenneth Collins, *Be Well!*

58 Mary Lowth (Reviewed by Prof Cathy Jackson), *Diseases and Different Ethnic Groups*, 3 December 2015, Certified by The Information Standard. https://patient.info/doctor/diseases-and-different-ethnic-groups (accessed 25 February 2019).

59 K. M. Goel, R. W. Logan, G. C. Arneil, E. M. Sweet, J. M. Warren, and R. A. Shanks, Florid and Subclinical Rickets among Immigrant Children in Glasgow, *Lancet*, 1976, pp. 1141–1145. Five percent of the Indian children had florid rickets, while there was none in a control group of Scottish, African and Chinese children. Mary Lowth (Reviewed by Prof Cathy Jackson), *Diseases and Different Ethnic Groups*, 3 December 2015, Certified by The Information Standard. https://patient.info/doctor/diseases-and-different-ethnic-groups (accessed 25 February 2019). Alison M. Bowes and Teresa M. Domokos, South Asian Women and Health Services: A Study in Glasgow, *New Community*, 9 (4), 1993, pp. 611–626, https://doi.org/10.1080/1369 183X.1993.9976391; K. M. Goel, S. Campbell, R. W. Logan, E. M. Sweet, A. Attenburrow, and G. C. Arneil, Reduced Prevalence of Rickets in Asian Children in Glasgow, *Lancet*, 318, 1981, pp. 405–407; M. G. Dunnigan, B. M. Glekin, J. B. Henderson, W. B. McIntosh, D. Sumner, and G. R. Sutherland, Prevention of Rickets in Asian Children: Assessment of the Glasgow Campaign, *British Medical Journal (Clinical Research Edition)*, 291, 1985, p. 239; K. M. Goel et al., Reduced Prevalence of Rickets in Asian Children in Glasgow, pp. 405–407.

60 K. M. Goel, S. Campbell, R. W. Logan, E. M. Sweet, A. Attenburrow, and G. C. Arneil, Reduced Prevalence of Rickets in Asian Children in Glasgow, *Lancet*, 318, 1981, pp. 405–407; M. G. Dunnigan, B. M. Glekin, J. B. Henderson, W. B. McIntosh, D. Sumner, and G. R. Sutherland, Prevention of Rickets in Asian Children: Assessment of the Glasgow Campaign, *British Medical Journal (Clinical Research Edition)*, 291, 1985, p. 239.

61 K. M. Goel et al., Reduced Prevalence of Rickets in Asian Children in Glasgow, pp. 405–407.

62 Two generations earlier, the novelist Lewis Grassic Gibbon and Scots poet Hugh MacDiarmid had written about the Jewish presence in the Gorbals, describing their clothes as 'unseemly' and their origins from 'alien suns'. Lewis Grassic Gibbon, Hugh MacDiarmid, on: Glasgow, *Scottish Scene*, 1934. The increasing ethnic population in Glasgow has led to many health initiatives; for example, the publication of David Walsh, *The Changing Ethnic Profiles of Glasgow and Scotland, and the Implications for Population Health* (Glasgow Centre for Population Health, Glasgow, 2017).

63 Stefano Bonino, Visible Muslimness in Scotland: Between Discrimination and Integration, *Patterns of Prejudice*, 49 (4), 2015, pp. 367–391.

64 'Definately': 'Definitely' pronounced with a Glasgow accent.

65 Stefano Bonino, Visible Muslimness in Scotland.

6

Clinical Topics

In general practice, any consultation could potentially take the practitioner down many different clinical pathways. While detailed knowledge of rare conditions would not be expected, the GP has to be able to recognise important symptoms and, where management is beyond the scope of general practice, refer the patient to the appropriate hospital department. Study participants described a very wide group of ailments which gives a broad indication of the GP workload.

GENERAL CLINICAL TOPICS

Participants recalled a wide range of clinical topics, especially relating to cardiovascular disease, kidney disease, lung diseases especially asthma, arthritis and the full range of infectious diseases. Through these clinical topics, I will show various aspects of the critical issues patients faced with access to their diagnosis and treatment.

Asthma is a common general practice respiratory problem, sometimes triggered by emotional or allergic factors. Up to the 1950s, the cause of asthma was usually thought to be stress-related, with some of the treatment in the hands of psychiatrists and psychoanalysts. Consequently, memories were of conflicts, such as these recollections from school or within the family. ZE recalled that 'The only illness I had was asthma that was brought on by my French teacher, 'cause I hated French at school. I hated the teacher'. ZNh remembered visiting her daughter after a phone call from a neighbour and needing the doctor to calm patient and mother. She said the following:

> To me, [she] was dying in the bed. That was the worst attack I'd ever seen her in. I thought she was gonna die. It was Dr Collins that told me, 'She can bring it on herself. See if she's in bother'—which she is quite a lot—she's a bad, bad manager. . . . Dr Collins said, 'It is a nervous asthma'—She was fighting fit the next day.

The next testimony concerns a patient, whose wife was angry at her husband's treatment by an out-of-hours doctor. She felt, with clearly every justification, that her husband needed immediate admission to hospital for oxygen, but the deputising doctor seems to have missed the signs, and her recollection was that he was giving

DOI: 10.1201/9781003369301-6

her the responsibility to take him to the hospital. I have no recollection of this event or of the quote attributed to me, but we have noted elsewhere that while events themselves were memorable for the patient, their attribution to a particular staff member is not always accurate. There were hospital doctors that worked during the night for the deputising services, but it is unlikely that anyone senior would have been one of them. However, if the scenario happened as related, the patient would have been satisfied with the idea that the complaint would have been relayed to Dr Ockrim and perhaps discussed at a later time.

> I don't think I had the oxygen at that time that's why [he] really needed the oxygen. [The doctor at home] said 'You just want me to shift him, well if you want him, you shift him'. Well, that wisnae [a] very nice doctor. . . . I said 'That's alright doctor, just go then. . . . I'll get him shifted'.
> He was very ill, and I came down [to the surgery] and spoke to your son and he said, 'I can't do anything because he's my senior, but I'll speak to my mother'. I said, 'I don't like to cause trouble, but I'm no' lettin' him away wi' it'.—After that I heard no more about it. I was only reporting what he had said to me and what he done to me which I didnae think was very nice.
>
> (LN)

Of course, not every illness can be resolved easily. The following is an account of a persistent problem which, despite many visits to the hospital for investigations and treatment, including surgical procedures, never seems to be resolved satisfactorily. At times, there seems to be a medical label for the condition, but at other times, the doctors seem to be at a loss and were casting widely around for guidance, leading to the patient's husband, as she says, 'really lost the head'. Uncertainty can lead to all sorts of speculation. The patient (LD) was worried that information was being withheld and that she might have had cancer. In the end, she just remarked, 'I get aboot wi' it. There's nae use in complainin' aboot it, is there?'

> I couldnae sleep and I was up during the night screaming wi' it. I couldnae walk and I couldnae get up and doon stairs. I was demented wi' it by this time. It was worse than it ever wis. . . . When I went back out to see the Orthopaedic Surgeon, he said he was very sorry, but it was back again. He said to be truthful he didnae know what it was. He gave it an awful funny name. It's something that's there but it's awful hard to get out. Well, I thought I had cancer. This was the second time he was saying he would discuss it with his colleagues and I definately thought I had cancer. He kept saying to me it was nothing nasty and I kept saying to myself, well if it's nothing nasty what' all this they've got to discuss.

It may seem hard to believe that treatment for the hyperacidity that is associated with gastric and duodenal ulcers involved surgery until the mid-1970s. Some of this surgery was the simpler vagotomy and pyloroplasty which involved cutting the vagus nerve which helped to reduce acid production and widened the exit route of food from the stomach. In many cases, the more radical partial gastrectomy was

performed. The outcome for sufferers of peptic ulcers first improved with the introduction of the histamine H2 receptor antagonist cimetidine in 1976 and later, the
proton-pump inhibitor omeprazole in 1988. The discovery in 1982 that ulcers were
caused by *Helicobacter pylori* bacteria led to the prescription of eradication therapy.
Not surprisingly, many of the memories of peptic ulcers came from the time when
the standard treatment was surgical. In this first memory, the patient felt that her
diagnosis had been missed on more than one occasion.

> I was being treated for stomach 'spasms.' That had gone on for two years.
> I am glad now that it happened the way it did because with it happening the
> way it did, I don't have an ulcer, and had it been known two years before that,
> I would have been getting treatment for it and I would have still had the ul-
> cer. . . . Before that happened, I wasn't well at all. It turned out it was this ulcer.
> [I] kept telling the medical profession that there was something the matter
> with me and they kept telling me there was nothing the matter with me. I had
> been taken into the hospital, three times, and got sent home. I must admit,
> I wasn't pleased at all. I felt I was going off my head, because I am telling them
> that I was ill—there was something the matter with me and they are keeping
> telling me, there's nothing wrong with you. [The ulcer] was in behind the
> duodenum. I said to [the surgeon], 'You told me there was nothing the matter
> with me.' He just smiled and shrugged his shoulders.
>
> (DQ)

Another participant who had experienced an ulcer some decades ago recalled
how, after a major operation removing most of his stomach, he still was unsure how
to tell the surgeon at a follow-up outpatient clinic how he felt:

> I cannae mind what year it was but they took me in and operated and took
> two thirds of my stomach away. I was off work for about six months. . . . I wis-
> nae actually vomiting, I was boaking[1]. So, I got word to come to the Bella-
> houston Dispensary. . . . and Mr Webster [the surgeon] was there wi' another
> couple of young students. I was frightened to tell him in case there was some-
> thing wrong. He said, 'How are you getting on?' I said, 'I don't know how to
> tell you this . . . every time I look at mince and potatoes now, I'm boaking at it'.
> He said, 'That's what I want . . . away you go home and have a fish supper and
> a pint of beer'. I said, 'Are you sure?' He said, 'Away you go home, and I don't
> want to see you again'. So that was me. I [now] eat like a horse.
>
> (ZI)

Hospital Complaints

Heart disease became the commonest of the degenerative diseases encountered in
general practice. Much of the recovery period after a heart attack involved advice on
diet, exercise and, above all, cigarette smoking. Consequently, when the communication between patient and staff was broken, for whatever reason, outcomes could be
affected, and advice was not always followed.

When I went into Intensive Care, the bed was broken, and I started complaining about the bed. I think this was why I got flung out the Southern without any real advice. OK, if I'd been given the advice, walking two miles in the morning and night, I probably wouldn't have been off my work for five months. OK, when they did put me on occupational therapy, I was one of the first people they tried with a heart attack and that's what got me back to work. They said, 'Cut out the eggs, butter and cheese.' I wasn't a heavy smoker—twenty a day which I still smoke. I gave up smoking when I was in hospital . . . eventually, I've just gone back to normal, as far as cigarettes are concerned.

(ZG)

The following participant described the story of her husband and his heart disease, during the mid-1970s. He was a successful businessman and was used to private hospital care. His views changed with the treatment he received for his heart attack in the Royal Infirmary, and he gave up his subscription for BUPA which had covered him for private hospital treatment.

he thought to himself, what can I do, I'm going to take a heart attack. . . . [A friend] took him to the Royal and when he got him to the Royal, he said that he wanted a private room, and they told him that they only did Health [Service]. He said, 'Well take me to the Victoria.' They said, 'You are going nowhere, but into Intensive Care.'

(QM)

One powerful memory related to an episode of arterial occlusion that was missed on more than one occasion by the casualty doctor who never expressed remorse over the incident which nearly cost the patient her leg:

On January [1977] I was taking [my daughter] to the nursery school, and I took there, terrific pains in both my legs. So, a friend carried on with [her] through the park. I hung on to the railings . . . it ended up, I came across to you and you had said to me, 'I honestly don't know what's wrong, because it's both your legs, but I want you to go down to the Southern General first thing in the morning'. So, you had given me a letter and I went away down. Unfortunately, I saw the most horrible man. He was a dreadful person and he told me that it was all my imagination, there was absolutely nothing wrong with me. . . . He had told me it was all in my mind. However, the pain, I didn't know where to put my legs and the pain was still in both my legs. So, this was the Thursday morning and you said, 'No, I'm not happy with his answer, go back again.' You shunted me away back to the Southern General. So down I went, and it was the same fellow who was still on, and he told me it was purely muscular, and it was all in my mind and it would pass.
   On the Saturday. . . . I noticed there was a discolouration purely at the calf of my leg, but nobody else saw it, except myself. So, I decided I would have to get a doctor. . . . So, I went away back again, and it was him I saw again. I said, 'Oh please, you'll have to help me.' Anyway, he went out and had a conversation

and he came back and said, 'Well, we'll admit you to Ward 15 since you're going to be so dramatic.' So, I got taken in to Ward 15. By this time, I was really in tears, because the pain was horrendous. So much so, that I must have been crying louder and by this time it was during the night. The night sister came up and said, 'You'll have to control yourself, you're disturbing other patients.' I said, 'Oh, please, could you help me?' She said, 'Let me see it.' She looked and said, 'Oh, good grief!' and she ran. Fortunately, Mr. McBain [the vascular surgeon] was on call and he came in. I could hear them at the end of my bed. He came up and he said, 'Well my dear, I'm afraid we'll have to get you to the theatre.' He said, 'I don't know where you've got a clot of blood and I don't know where it's lying, but all probability, your leg will be amputated.' I fainted. Anyway, I remember when I came round, I was wrapped in tin foil. He came up to me and said that he was delighted to tell me that the clot, which was four inches long had lodged at the top of my groin, but my toes were in danger, so I had a blood bank feeding into an artery.

(FW)

When Dr Ockrim asked about the doctor who had refused to recognise her symptoms at the beginning and whether he had apologised, she said the following:

the young fellow couldn't look at me. No [apology]. I think he was so embarrassed.[2] I wanted to say to him, just try and be a little more tactful the next time. He just slithered at the back. It was a bit embarrassing, but then I thought, I hadn't done anything. I only wanted help.

(EX)

EX also recalled that practice procedures had changed. Instead of a practice visit for repeat medication, she said that she hardly went to the surgery now, and she would just 'use my repeat prescription card—when Dr Ockrim was there, I would never have been allowed to do that. I remember you phoned me and told me to come along'.

Another incident recalled by a participant concerned her mother's admission to Shieldhall Hospital, which, by the 1950s, served as the geriatric unit of the Southern General Hospital. Geriatric wards usually had a mixture of patients with disabilities of old age, including dementia as well as physical problems, often following a stroke. Patients who were mentally alert often resented being in the same ward as those who had advanced dementia.

I remember one time she went in [to hospital] and I was quite angry, because they sent her to Shieldhall Hospital. She shouldn't have been sent there really, because she was alright in her mind. When she went there, they used to mix her dinner up, like the poor souls that were there. They took her money off her . . . and I remember her saying, 'They won't give me my paper money.' I would say, 'Why?' She would say 'I'm not fit to look after it or something'. She was only there a day, and she was going right down so I went to see about it and one doctor said he had nothing to do with her going there. . . . So,

I went to see the Matron of the Southern General and she said to me that she should not be there and for me to write a letter to the Medical Board about this. Then I seen the other man, the Superintendent and he wasn't all that nice about it at first.[3] I saw the Deputy Superintendent and he was such a nice person. He agreed with Matron.

I eventually had a row down there and I had to get the ambulance. I demanded to take my mother home. The ambulance were having a dispute that day. I said, 'I'll take a taxi, if you give me medical staff with me to get her home'. So, I ended up with a taxi and with a nurse. . . . However, I got my mother home, and she came on after that. My brother-in-law wrote this letter to the Medical Board and they invited him and I down to a conference, have our lunch, have a conference with them.

(LNf)

Misattributed Diagnosis

The classic symptoms of the high level of blood sugar include increased thirst and urination, but the longer-term complications can include cardiovascular and kidney diseases, retinopathy, neuropathy and skin ulceration. The prevalence of diabetes has been rising and is currently estimated to affect around 8% of the adult population, with a significant proportion not yet diagnosed. Most patients have Type 2 diabetes, where insulin resistance develops and is associated with excess body weight; this can usually be treated with weight loss and oral medication. Around 10% have Type 1 diabetes, where insulin-producing pancreatic beta cells are lost due to an autoimmune process, and patients require insulin injections.

One participant claimed that her diabetes was diagnosed by the practice manager, Nanette Aitken, who strongly denies the account, commenting that she would never have acted in this way, and it seems more likely that the doctor would have requested the urine sample.

Oh, I'll tell you what it was, I was feeling so ill and this particular day I thought, I've got to go down and see Dr [David] Collins. I did that and I realised that before I would reach the surgery I could collapse. I knew how bad I felt, and when I went in Nanette said to me, 'Whatever is wrong with you? I don't like to say but you're looking dreadful today'. I said, 'I feel terrible'. She said, 'See me when you come out after seeing the doctor'. So, I did, and I think it was Dr Collins. I told him how I felt. He said, 'Do you feel as though you're not walking well?' I said, 'Yes I do'. He said, 'I'll give you this and come back again if you think it's not helping'. So, I went out and told Nanette. Of course, she had had experience through her own mother of being diabetic. She said to me, 'Let me see what doctor has given you'. She said, 'Did you take a sample of your urine?' I said, 'No, I didn't think about that'. She said, 'Well give me one now and I'll test it for you, and I'll take it in and see doctor'. So, I did. When she came through after testing it, I said, 'Well?'. Right away I knew. I said, 'Is it sugar?' She said, 'Loaded, absolutely loaded'. So, when I went in to see Dr Collins again, I sat down and he said, 'I'm very pleased I got this today. . . . I'll have a specimen of your blood and I'll have it tested somewhere and I'll find out just what's the matter'.

(LN1)

This was not the only recollection of a diagnosis by the practice manager. In another story, the patient's recollection is that the diagnosis of pregnancy was given to the patient by the practice manager, Nanette Aitken. Nanette again explained that she would never give any patient medical information and that the scenarios as described could not have happened:

Then it dawned on me that I hadnae seen an illness[4]. It was then I came along, and I told you and you sent a specimen away. Well, when I went back for the result of the specimen it was Nanette and quite laughingly, she said, 'Well would you like to be pregnant, or would you like to be feeling the way you are?' I said, 'What!' She said, 'I'm telling you you're pregnant'. I said, 'You are joking'. Well, I cried the whole way home.

(DD)

Chronic renal failure is manageable, firstly, with medication and diet; then secondly, dialysis (usually haemodialysis); and finally, for some, transplantation, but the process from diagnosis to transplant can be long in time and arduous for patient and family. Successful haemodialysis, which removes waste products such as creatinine and urea, developed only around 1960, beginning as a hospital procedure. Successful transplantation only became available from the 1960s as therapies to counter tissue rejection became available. The first kidney transplant in Glasgow was performed at the Royal Infirmary in 1968, but subsequent transplants were carried out at the Western Infirmary. In 1972, a unit was established at Stobhill Hospital which focussed on supporting home haemodialysis patients and their carers.[5]

The following illustrates the story from the patient's viewpoint while showing the strains the illness places on the family. From the beginning of dialysis to the final stage of transplantation, freeing the patient from the dependency on dialysis and the frequent feelings of helplessness that it engenders, there were problems with how the family were dealt with all the way through.

While they were doing all sorts of tests [at Belvedere Hospital], they discovered something wrong with the kidneys . . . and the results showed some scarring and that I had a bit of a kidney problem was all I was told at the time . . . five years [later], I was very tired and there was this taste in my mouth. . . . I went to my local doctor, and he sent me back to the Royal. They discovered there was deterioration in the kidneys. . . . It was three years later before I needed dialysis.

I was one of the longest on the waiting list for a transplant. . . . I just kept saying, well a kidney will come at some time, but we just pushed it to the back of our minds, and it was something we never really thought about after so long. We got a phone call in July, and I have now had a transplant. . . .

It was a four-hour operation. The next day when I came round, everything seemed to be working and I was let out of hospital after a week. The kidney has been working for ten weeks now. I have been back at work for the last two weeks, and I am feeling great. [My skin] is starting to clear up and I have a lot more energy.

(AK)

If things had been difficult for the patient, they had often been fraught for the wife and extended family. She explained as follows:

I felt my whole world had just caved in. How could my husband to be so ill? I just didn't know how I would cope with it. Other people have got burdens they have to deal with, and this was just something that had happened to us and if we didn't get up and get on with it then it would appear more drastic than it was.

I felt as if the hospital just put him out after a week [following the transplant]—it was dreadful. The service in the hospital—it wasn't their fault. There was lack of money, lack of funds. Two or three days after having his transplant, I went up to visit and he was sitting in a day ward and was still connected to tubes and catheters and different things and he was in that day ward the whole day, because they never had a bed for him. . . . After a week he got home, and I didn't think he should have got home. He got bed rest here and better service here, but I was dead apprehensive when he came home.

(FK)

Sharing the Diagnosis

Multiple sclerosis is a disease, one of relapses and remissions, where the coverings of nerve cells in the brain and spinal cord are damaged. This damage disrupts the ability of parts of the nervous system to transmit signals, resulting in a range of signs and symptoms, including physical, mental and sometimes psychiatric problems. Frequent symptoms may include double vision, blindness in one eye, muscle weakness and problems with sensation or coordination. Many patients exhibit a mild euphoria which may aid acceptance of the condition, but there was a reluctance to tell patients the diagnosis until the condition was definitely established. One participant told the doctor that she was 'awful worried' about her daughter who was having frequent falls. She was referred to the neurology clinic at the Southern General for diagnostic tests:

[My daughter] said she knew what was wrong with her before she went in. She said to Dr Grieve, 'I know what's wrong with me'. She told her she had multiple sclerosis. When she came out, she was crying. She said, 'Mum, I'm not crying'. She says, 'I'm crying with happiness, because I know what's wrong with me'. She said, 'I know I'm going to fight it because it's no' gonnae get the better of me. . . . They don't have a cure for it, but I'm quite reconciled to the fact that I've got it but I'm not going to let it get me down and sit about'.

(GT)

Another participant described the care she gave her mother, who was severely disabled with multiple sclerosis. She explained how her mother was wheelchair-bound, and they moved her bed to the living room. It took a long time for the diagnosis to be established, as the daughter recalled the following:

> Now I remember her saying to me, she was about 37 and she didn't know what was wrong with her and she had . . . a late baby and I think this is what brought this on. At that time, she didn't know it was that. I would say it was about 48 when they discovered she had MS.
>
> (LNf)

Surgical Procedures

This first story concerns a patient who had emigrated many years earlier but, dissatisfied with her treatment in America, decided to return to her sisters in Glasgow, following a colostomy operation in the United States. She had lost a lot of weight but had been told that the condition was not malignant. The treatment in Scotland proved to be curative, and the surgeon from the Victoria Infirmary did not mince words with the surgeon in America.

> [Her husband] kept saying if she had such great faith in the doctors over here, he'd better get her over. So, it was arranged that she was to fly over here. . . . Anyway, Dr Collins came and he. . . . I may be wrong, but I think he had a friend who was a surgeon from the Victoria Infirmary. Dr Collins got him to come to check [her] over, at the house.[6] Immediately he said to [her], 'They've left you in a dreadful state: the operation should have been reversed.' . . . She had about three or four different operations in and out . . . [over] about 6 weeks. It was truly amazing the difference in her eventually. After a spell she went back to America. When she went back everybody—they couldn't believe it. . . . However, she went to her own doctor and her surgeon, and this particular doctor looked, and she said, 'Don't you see a difference doctor?' He said, 'Oh yes, I remember you, your doctor in Scotland wrote and called me a butcher.'
>
> (LN)

Not all surgical interventions were as successful as this, and the complications of surgery could leave a lasting effect on the family members. In the first of these testimonies, an observation is made that her brother had an operation and was 'ripped open without giving him anything'. The illness is described in graphic terms, though it seems hard to understand as a purely medical account.

> Well, my mother wasn't in favour of hospitals because I had a brother who had taken peritonitis and took a cerebral haemorrhage in the brain, and they took him back to the hospital. . . . They ripped him open without giving him anything. I can always remember that. She never had any faith in the Royal. . . . That's when they opened him up. It ended up, he ended up in the

Western with spinal fever. He was blind, he was speechless, and he was para-lysed. It was so heart breaking to see him . . . the other day they sent for her, and they said he had a treble haemorrhage of the brain, and they moved him to Killearn [Neurosurgery Department]. They operated but the haemorrhage went over the brain, and he died.

(LI)

One participant described how her daughter was admitted to hospital with pro-fuse rectal bleeding with a sequence of events that led to a specialist in London who was performing a new procedure called an Ivalon sponge rectopexy.[7]

I called the doctor. She [my daughter] was admitted that night to the South-ern General. . . . She was in quite a while, and they couldn't find the source. Eventually Mr Tankel [the surgeon][8] sent for us himself and he admitted that she was having substantial bleeding, but he couldn't find the source. He was bringing in a second opinion. I felt reassured. He was bringing in a second opinion because he could not find the source. His words were, 'I'm a consultant surgeon, I'm not a specialist. I've dabbled in fields I shouldn't have, and I've been successful.' He said, 'She's too young . . . and I feel she should be put into the hands of specialists.' He said, 'I'm afraid it'll have to be London.'

(IK)

The final recollection here describes the following of a patient with such chronic constipation that eventually, major surgery had to be carried out. The patient recalled that the surgeon indicated that this would be his first time car-rying out the procedure, in around 1982, though he was able to publish a study of his experience with the operation in 1987.[9] After many investigations, the first surgeon said that he thought that 'it was a psychological problem' and that she should be referred to a psychiatrist. She disagreed with the suggestion that the condition was psychological and eventually had an operation which had to be repeated some years later.

from there I went back to Dr Collins and Dr Collins agreed with myself that I didnae need a psychiatrist and he asked me if I was willing to give it one more go, and he sent me to the Western. I went to the Western, to the Gastro-Intestinal Centre and they took me in for a week to the Gardner In-stitute. After a week of tests and x-rays, Dr Birnie asked me if I would take the chance of going through the operation and to relieve the pain. I was quite happy to do it.

They would refer me to Peebles-Brown at Gartnavel General and he took me in for a week and he x-rayed me and done all sorts of tests and things. He said that I would need this operation, but this would be the first time that he was actually performing the operation. . . . My bowel went fine for about eighteen months to two years after that.

(LH)

This recollection is of a participant who developed thyrotoxicosis (an over-active thyroid). Listening to her account the symptoms of thyrotoxicosis seem so obvious that one wonders why it took so long for the penny to drop.

I said, 'Oh, don't tell me I've got multiple sclerosis [like] my mother [who] used to start out at the hedge and land out on the pavement'. I would get up off this chair and I would stagger . . . so I went down to the surgery, and it was Dr Russell, I think I seen. He sent me to the Southern General and I was there a number of times before they discovered.

There was three doctors and they all took me and gave me the same examination and then when they were finished with that, they went away and had a consultation about it. Dr Kirkwood came back and said to me, 'Well, we have got a bed upstairs for you. It's the only one we've got, and we have kept it for you because we have all decided that you've got an over-active thyroid. I'd never heard of that either'.

(LNf)

Infectious Diseases: Memories were especially strong in relation to tuberculosis and the stigma which accompanied it. This association with stigma has already been described in the previous chapter. In the aftermath of coronavirus, it is hard to say that infectious disease is something from the past, but the main childhood illnesses of diphtheria, whooping cough, mumps and measles now all have effective vaccines, as do Covid-19, influenza and tuberculosis. Memories were long enough to include diseases such as diphtheria and smallpox, no longer seen today. One of the interviewees had developed diphtheria in 1929, along with six of her friends, and they were all admitted and put into a ward in Shieldhall Hospital. Management at the time was with the anti-toxin, made from the plasma of horses immunised against diphtheria. The therapy was not without side effects, but as diphtheria was a significant cause of morbidity and mortality, it was an essential treatment. The condition became less common with the introduction of a diphtheria vaccine. IT recalled that 'It was my throat to begin with and glands and ears and I reported it and a swab was taken and that was that'. So she was given 'so many units of the serum'.

ZI mentioned that his mother had had diphtheria when she was a child and needed a tracheostomy. He started training in 1931 to be a sanitary inspector and remembered this:

Diphtheria was rife, scarlet fever was rife, mastoids were rife. I had two young cousins die from mastoids. It was particularly tragic for my family because one of them was called after my mother and she died and then there was a little boy born and he was called after my father and the two of them died of mastoids.

When it was a case of any of these illnesses, we used to be sent to test the drains—smoke test them and there was leakages all over the place and the back courts used to be flooded with choked drains and you would see all the children playing in them. You had to be very hardy to survive in these days.

A rare infection is Legionnaires' disease. The interviewee contracted the illness while in Spain where the diagnosis was never mentioned. It was not mentioned to her either despite several weeks in hospital in Glasgow. She had to be admitted to the Southern General from Glasgow Airport and then transferred to Ruchill Hospital where it took almost a month of treatment before she was fully recovered. It was only shortly before discharge when the consultant, accompanied by some medical students, passed by her bed, and she heard him say, 'Now Mrs N went to Majorca a healthy woman and came back with Legionnaires' Disease'. 'That was the first I heard it. I nearly took a heart attack because I never knew that (LNf)'.

Scarlet fever is a streptococcal infection and symptoms include sore throat, fever, headache and a characteristic rash. Complications of the infection include acute rheumatic fever, glomerulo-nephritis and arthritis. It has become more common again in Britain in recent years as antibiotic resistance has increased. Memories related to measures taken at home are as follows:

> My sister had scarlet fever, and, in those days, they were taken away right away, you know, and the house was fumigated with the candle that they burn.
>
> (CT)

Others were more concerned by the memories of hospital visiting which restricted access of children to their parents:

> I was in hospital for scarlet fever. I was in Belvidere. . . . I remember, when you go to Belvidere, your parents weren't tae get in then. When you went in there was a waiting room and a long wall with windows across the top. The nurses, whoever came to these windows, and you gave them your whatever, for your child and the parents spoke to whoever was above.
>
> (LI)

Cancer: The diagnosis of cancer was the most feared by participants in the oral history study. Although, the average general practitioner will only look after two such patients to the end of life in a year. In addition, home care will be provided for four more patients before the final event in hospice or hospital, an Editorial in the *Journal of the Royal College of General Practitioners* in 1986 considered it was one of hardest topics to discuss.[10]

I will show, through the memories of cancer within the family, how these recollections shed light on the relationships with doctors and other health care workers and how these relationships changed over time as society became more open about the diagnosis. Regarded as a death sentence, we were not permitted as medical students in the late 1960s to mention the word 'cancer' in front of patients, using euphemisms instead. This reluctance to tell the truth to patients persisted into more recent times. Patients, or their families, would return from the local chest clinic telling me that they did not have cancer, while the letter from the clinician indicated otherwise. Interpreting the exact words that had been used at the hospital, it was clear that the consultant had been using language as a subterfuge to avoid telling the patient the truth.[11] As the following shows, it was the family that received the diagnosis:

> Dr Monie, and he done the bronchoscope. We went down to collect her that day, and we were told [the diagnosis] within the next two or three days

and I refused to go—I didnae want to know and they told us then—eight weeks, which was—It was the most horrible thing, and I wouldn't accept the fact.

(ZNg)

Told that the patient had only months to live, she survived for more than two years, staying at home to the end, having refused treatment other than pain relief and relying on practice and family support. Properly handled, home care can provide the patient and the family with the support that they need through the hard times that are consequent with a final illness.

Dr O'Neill was great, and he explained what was going to happen. If we needed—no matter what we needed, we were to phone the surgery at any time—day or night. We couldnae have asked for a better doctor than Dr O'Neill and the care that he gave my mother. . . . She looked forward to dying and she looked forward to that boy coming. I mean, she would make an effort to wash her face, comb her hair, spray her deodorant.

(ZNg)

The idea of an incurable disease was hard for many clinicians to accept, and textbooks counselled doctors not to give patients the diagnosis of cancer, which would deprive them of hope. The concept of terminal care was virtually unknown before the 1960s.[12] It was left to pioneers like Dame Cecily Saunders, who created the hospice movement and began to focus on a patient-centred approach with a better approach to pain relief.

I think she [my mother] really knew all along [that she had cancer.] I think she knew she would never come out of hospital. Probably she knew before we were ready to accept it. . . . Well, after the first operation they said that there were some cancerous cells, which probably didn't have a great impact on us. We didn't really realise the extent of the cancer.

(KNk)

The following recollection concerns a patient who was diagnosed with lung cancer in 1963 but got the impression, which was never corrected, that she had TB. Non-smokers can develop lung cancer through passive inhalation of tobacco smoke or other pollutants.

She [my wife] never smoked and didn't drink. You were the person who attended her.

It came from the one lung to the other lung, and it spread round the heart. . . . I would say, from the diagnosis of having cancer, they said it would be nine months and it was nine months. She was sent down for x-ray and they instilled in her the idea that it could be TB. They put her to Mearnskirk. They let it be that she could live with the idea that it was TB. Yes. She died thinking that.

(VF)

Yes, she had cancer but it just wisnae diagnosed till it wis too late. Actually, at the beginning, she didnae know what she had. It was pains in her back as far as she knew and when you've got pains in your back, in those days, it was pains in your back. You never for a minute suspected that you had cancer in your womb, in these days.

(KNa)

A study carried out in the West of Scotland a couple of years after the project finished indicated changing attitudes to information about cancer, as almost all cancer patients interviewed wanted information about their illness, the diagnosis, their chance of cure and the possible side effects of treatment.[13] A substantial minority of British doctors were avoiding telling patients that they have cancer, through a sense of unease about discussing serious illness and dying, feeling that knowledge of the diagnosis will depress and alarm patients, and will impair their quality of life.

Some studies have shown that protecting patients from the truth may be counterproductive. While emotional distress is transiently greater when patients are told the diagnosis, there are positive effects concerning coping, compliance, tolerance of treatment, planning for future occasion and communication with physicians.[14] This attitude to avoid telling the patient the diagnosis was sometimes accompanied by telling family members the truth, creating a barrier between patient and relatives. Others, however, have indicated that the anxiety and depression generated by a cancer diagnosis should not be underestimated. One study carried out in Glasgow and published in the *Journal of Epidemiology and Community Health* indicated that severe depressive illness is significantly associated with a lung cancer diagnosis.[15] This may be, the authors suggested, due to personality factors, including previous psychiatric history, the presence of metastases, not receiving a specific treatment, lack of a social support system, lack of information and poor coping behaviour mechanisms. Consequently, proper patient understanding was essential to allow measures of psychological adjustment before and after treatment so that appropriate supportive care, for example, psychiatric consultation, can be provided. The hospice movement began with an attempt to meet the need for adequate pain control in cancer patients but gradually extended into providing hospices for a holistic approach to terminal care as well as supporting patients at home.[16]

While death rates from lung cancer have been falling, the reduction was greater in more affluent areas.[17] Postcode sectors in Scotland that were categorised as deprived in 1981 were relatively more deprived at the time of the 1991 census. The Scottish Cancer Therapy Network (SCTN), which documents clinical practice and the use of evidence-based clinical guidelines, also found that patient lung cancer, from deprived communities, are at a disadvantage when it comes to treatment and survival.[18] Indeed, SCTN has strongly recommended that such patients should be managed by a lung cancer specialist. While general practices strive to provide for their cancer patients and their terminal care when required, some studies indicated the practical problems when membership of the primary care practice team is augmented by cancer specialist nurses. Margaret Kindlen pointed to such issues as 'role identity, role conflict and ambiguity, and resistant attitudes' in her research, also pointing to matters related to nurse specialisation, professional teamwork and information sharing between patients, families and professionals.[19]

I had a feeling that she knew [she had cancer]. Only once, she said, 'I don't like my colour, I think there's something deeper than what they're telling me.'

(LNl)

She knew she was going to die. She refused to accept the fact. No-one was to mention the word cancer—no one, not even Dr O'Neill, not even the priest and no one was to mention cancer . . . but she wanted—if she was going to die, she wanted to die in her own home, with her own family and we gave her her wish—I felt, my mother kept her dignity. To me, if my mother had lost her dignity, she would have died before she died.

(ZNg)

The greater readiness to inform cancer patients of the diagnosis has to be tempered with an understanding of each patient, their psychological make-up and their response to hard news. Sometimes the condition progressed so rapidly that patients and their families struggled to cope with its emotional impact.

My aunt was told, in the Western that she had cancer. She didn't want to believe it. She never told us she had cancer. I seen my aunt bottling this up. In one particular ward in the Beatson [cancer hospital] most of the women in the ward had lost their hair and she turned round and said to me one night, this is the wrong ward for me. . . . She said, this is for people who are terminally ill. Then she was advised to go to a home in Duntocher—a hospice. She was in the hospital at the time, and I told a wee white lie. I went down myself one night and she broke. She said, 'I don't want to go in there'. I said, 'There's nothing wrong with it'. I said, 'You only go in there to try and get yourself better'. She said, 'Do you really believe that?' I said, 'Of course, I believe it'.

(AF)

The concern about cancer could lead patients just to accept treatment without questioning:

I didn't ask [what was wrong]. Not being in that frame of mind, I didn't worry, as long as it wasn't cancer.

(LNa)

Sometimes, with cancer, it is hard to pinpoint the primary lesion early on. The following daughter's account is of a patient whose first symptoms suggested a lung lesion and then possibly bladder disease before a spinal tumour was diagnosed after a body scan. She recalled that she 'had a funny idea that it was a cancerous tumour'.

[My father] hadnae been feeling well and we kept saying, you better go to the doctor and see about it. . . . We knew there must be something wrong. I said to him I would phone the doctor. Dr Collins came out and said, 'I think we'll have to put you in for further investigations'. . . . They took him to neurosurgical and did all these tests on him and then they discovered he had a tumour in the spine. They done a body scan. I asked to see the doctor. They said it was a tumour, but they didn't know what kind of tumour it was. I had a funny idea that it was a cancerous tumour.

Well, he's never asked me if I know [the diagnosis], but I've been dropping hints. I said to him the other week—because the doctor spoke to me. He said, 'I'm sorry to give you the bad news, but it's not very good. I think your dad is going to eventually just pass away.'

(GH)

Breast lumps also carry a great deal of anxiety, although many swellings, as in the first story here, are quite benign, though still requiring careful testing before the patient can be fully reassured.

Oh well, just a cyst I had on my breast. You sent me to the David Elder [Infirmary]. I don't know how many years ago that wis. In fact, you gave me the letter to go the next day. I always mind 'cause it was quick and I seen this doctor in the David Elder and he put it down to a cyst. . . . He more or less assured me that it was a cyst. It turned out it was anyway, and I was only in for three days.

(BE)

In another memory, a participant describes how his wife had breast cancer alongside episodes of anxiety and depression during and after the treatment despite being reassured that the cancer therapy had been successful.

Other than that, she enjoyed good health until this depression set in. We don't know [why] really. Of course, she had to get one of her breasts off for cancer. . . . Sir Robert Wright, I think was the consultant she saw[20]. He did the operation right away. He took a test, and he said it was malignant and the breast would have to come off. He sent for me one day. He said, 'She is taking it very good and she's happy and accepting it'. He said, 'It's up to you now that she stays that way'. She was great until she came out. [When she came home] I was a wee bit disappointed in that. I thought someone would be round. She wouldnae let me go in when she was undressed, but the wound was leaking, and she was having to dress it herself in the morning. I thought they should have sent somebody to help her. We should have got in contact. I should have done it myself. I think they warned her [in the hospital] that it would leak, and they gave her dressings. Aye, after that he sent her over to the Western for radium treatment.

She got the all-clear and she said she hadn't to go back for a year. She did worry at times. Well on the surface she didnae seem to bother. She didnae seem to feel any different. I cannae say it made any difference to her. She didnae like that sort of talk. If I tried to get on that subject she would say, 'Oh, don't talk about that.'

(ZR)

To begin with she went to the Victoria, and they knew she was a diabetic. She had this wee ulcer in her tongue, and they used to put gentian violet and something else on it and they would never take to do with her because I think she was a diabetic. This doctor, after many years said, 'Right! I'll tell you what to do. You bring her to my place at the Beatson and I'll give her an examination.' So, they came to the conclusion. 'I don't have to think any harder' he said, 'I'm quite sure what it is. Unfortunately,' he said, 'it's too far gone. . . . We'll do what we can.'

They took out all her teeth and cut her tongue and then they took away the glands. Then they took away the muscle. I used to feel so vexed. I just thought to myself, what they're putting her through and the time she's got. . . . I think [her husband] got to the stage that he wanted them to do anything just to keep her. They put radium in her tongue. When I went up, they warned me before I went in. He said, 'Now before you go in, don't show any emotion because she really isn't pleasant to look at.' She had radium needles right the way down and she couldn't speak, but she could hear, and she would write down, 'The birds sound beautiful today, I've been listening all morning to them.' I used to think, 'How can you think like that?—the state you're in.'

(LNl)

The fear of cancer and the reluctance by many clinicians to be open with their patients led to suspicions by families that a cancer diagnosis was being withheld. One patient, who was concerned about her sister, explained that she was not satisfied with her discussion with her sister's specialist and his diagnosis of diverticulitis:

Well, I thought it was [cancer]. I thought it was a possibility it could be. I might be miss-judging [the surgeon], but I felt that he was just—as though there was nothing between the ears. It might have been right, but at the time, I took it with a pinch of salt. I thought there was more to it.

(IU)

One participant made no reference to religion during the interview, but his mother's terminal nursing care, in which I was closely involved, had an unexpected and almost spiritual quality:

I remember talking to Dr Kenneth Collins about it and asking him to give her more pain-relieving drugs and he explained what would happen. He said that she would become delirious. I said, 'I didn't care.' Get it over with is my attitude. He didn't see it quite that way. Strangely enough, but those last few weeks for me were quite special, I got very close to my mother then and also, I found it quite, in a sense, exhilarating, because I had never seen a death before like that. There was something quite pleasant about it, it was strange. Something about the peace—she seemed to have a lot of peace at the end. . . . It was a great understanding of what death was about, I suppose, and I'm quite content about it.

(ZT)

The diagnosis of cancer, a generation ago, was usually seen as a death sentence, though good results were already seen in breast and some other cancers. With improving treatments and a greater awareness of the disease, there was less of a reluctance to speak about the condition openly. With dedicated cancer care nurses and better programmes of pain relief provided by district nurses came a greater acceptance of home care in the terminal phase.

OBSTETRICS AND GYNAECOLOGY

The oral history study covers memories of childbirth over forty years. The era begins with most births taking place at home and continues with the increasing medical-isation of childbirth so that it is now uncommon for any births at all to take place outside hospital. During these years, the involvement of general practitioners in intra-partum care declined. Some GPs, like Dr Ockrim, continued their obstetric work in nursing homes or hospital GP units, but even this gradually declined. The case against GP or midwife-led deliveries follows studies which show that there is a high rate of transfer to specialist services which cannot be predicted in advance.[21] In 2011, the National Childbirth Trust briefing included the following statement:

> All pregnant women should be able to make choices about their planned place of birth. There should be sufficient provision of midwifery-led services, based on a social model of care, to meet the demand in all areas.[22]

However local budgetary issues severely curtailed choice.

In this section, we will examine the patient attitudes to GP care of pregnancy, follow the changes that occurred and understand what was important to mothers. Many participants had concluded that home was the better option, and greater acceptance of hospital deliveries only came with the provision of upgraded facilities or even new buildings for maternity care.

> Better [with a home delivery]. Well, I can only go back to the conditions of the Southern General at that time. They had two wards, and two toilets . . . the new Maternity [Unit]—that was the most wonderful thing that ever hap-pened in Govan. It's sheer luxury. They would rather go in there now, as have them at home. They get peace. . . . But in the Southern years ago, I wouldnae wish that on anybody.
>
> (FS)

> Stobhill [Hospital], I think is very run down. . . . Even my maternity treatment—it was OK having the baby, but things like the ward—You were going for a bath, and you had to make sure that you had thoroughly scrubbed the bath before going into it. You were finding yourself wiping things down before using them. It was dirty. I think there should have been a cleaner in there at the start of the day gutting it and it wasn't always the case, and bins weren't always emptied
>
> (FK)

Nursing staff did not tolerate difficult behaviour. One participant remembered that the woman in the next bed was smacked because she had been screaming. The sister said the following:

'You're upsetting everybody else. You've already had three kids and thae other lassies have no' had babies and you're frightening them—behave yourself!' So, she got scudded.[23]

(HNa)

In recent years, paternalistic attitudes in the wards changed. Even patients that had babies a few years apart noticed a significant change. For older patients, who had always accepted authority with simple obedience, there was the beginning of understanding that some procedures were optional and maybe even questionable. Linda McMahon recalled the following:

I think when my oldest was born there was a kind of rigid routine in the hospital. You had to do this, you had to do that. You weren't allowed to pick up the baby. It never occurred to me after she was born that I could pick her up any time I wanted. I felt she still belonged to the hospital. I picked her up to feed her and change her and I put her back down and that was it. I didn't pick her up because I wanted to. By the time the youngest was born it was a far more relaxed atmosphere and the nurses would sit on the bed and chat to you, and you would call them by their first name instead of Sister Starched Apron giving you a row because you weren't eating your sprouts. I saw quite a difference and that was only a difference of nine years.

(Linda McMahon)

Well, I'm older and I know a lot more—then you kept your mouth shut. You did as you were told. They came along with a tray of castor oil and orange juice. . . . I was feeling sick taking it. She went to the next bed, and she refused it, and I was the only one in the ward that took it. I was the first to get it and I didn't realise you could refuse it. Now, I think with experience, you do question things, and you say, 'Well is that right?'

(BC)

One participant felt distressed with the advice given by her hospital obstetrician, and she left the hospital antenatal clinic and made straight to Cessnock Street to be reassured by Dr Ockrim.

I think it really was the way I expected it to be, other than one doctor, I think she was a registrar and I had heard stories about her. Well, not very good ones. . . . She had measured me with an inch tape and hummed and hawed and hadn't appeared happy, but she hadn't said anything, and she just said, 'Come back in a month.' . . . She obviously was thinking there was something not right, but she hadn't said anything.

When this particular doctor came round the ward when [my daughter] was born, she said something about 'Well it's definitely a very small baby, I'm just going to underline this'. I thought this was really childish. She was just trying to show me that she was right. [My daughter] was fine and she's not exactly a small child now.

(KNk)

Home Deliveries

When the NHS began, general practitioners were responsible for most of their patients' deliveries. Around half were conducted at home, and others in the private nursing homes around Glasgow, but by 1975, virtually every birth took place in hospital. Major changes in the delivery of maternity care followed Sir John Peel's Report of 1970 which stated that every woman should have access to hospital care when giving birth.[24] The Report's aim was to reduce maternal and infant mortality, but the move had a profound effect on domiciliary midwifery. It was becoming difficult for general practitioners to get enough of a caseload to maintain their expertise, as participation during labour was limited by other commitments. The Royal College of Obstetricians and Gynaecologists reported in 1982 that 'it is not possible to predict with accuracy which labours will be uncomplicated', and they hoped 'few, if any, pregnant women will be delivered at home'.[25] Bull considered in the 1980s that the general practitioner accoucheur will still have a role, but heroics in their field will no longer be appropriate.[26]

An *Occasional Paper* of the Royal College of General Practitioners (RCGP) in 1995 noted that in maternity care, the decisions about specialist care have come from the hospital sector, and the views of general practitioners have been marginalised.[27] The *Occasional Paper* supported a GP role in care before and after birth but indicated that any intra-partum participation by the GP was only in support of the residual element of domiciliary midwives.

These views were widely accepted, though other voices, such as Campbell and MacFarlane, questioned the safety claims and said that many women felt that the hospital was an alien environment and that they were more comfortable at home.[28] Patients had seen many advantages in having a home delivery with a family support network around them and attendance by the now familiar figure of the family doctor. While general practitioners were expected to be available to patients even during the delivery, most doctors were happy to leave things to the local midwives and be guided by them if complications occurred necessitating hospital admission. The Central Board for Midwives in Scotland (CBMS) was dominated by general practitioners and obstetricians until 1983, reflecting the difficult relationship between GPs and midwives.[29]

One of the interviewees was Sister Margaret French, who had first been a community midwife before working at the St Francis Nursing Home and then at the Southern General Hospital. She said that 'when the doctor delivers patients, there's a kind of bond . . . they feel very secure with their own doctor' but also acknowledged many GPs were happy to leave things to the midwives. Midwives would often spend many hours with their patients, while general practitioners, who had to juggle other commitments, would often need to confine their time to a short period of assessment and then return in time for the delivery.

An oral history exploration of the experiences of Scottish midwives was conducted by Lindsay Reid and published in 2008. The traditional unqualified birth assistant, the howdie, commonly found in rural areas, was still operating in Glasgow as late as the 1940s.[30] The recollections of more than twenty midwives covers much of the same period as the women in this study were undergoing their pregnancies and childbirth.[31] Midwife grievances included the need for a general practitioner to authorise the call for the emergency flying squad.[32] It was also recognised that studies of maternal mortality showed that deaths occurred at twice the rate in the more middle-class homes served by the general practitioners than in the poorer households where the midwives conducted the deliveries.[33]

Lindsay Reid described the remorseless drive to medicalise childbirth which has marginalised midwives and has led to the belief that only hospital deliveries can be considered 'safe'.[34] Major developments in the conduct of labour had also made a substantial difference to the perceived benefits of hospital delivery until the need for district midwives all but disappeared. Questions were then raised: has medicalisation gone too far?[35]

Dr Ockrim and Obstetrics

Dr Ockrim entered general practice following hospital training in obstetrics and gynaecology, and she had undertaken a brief course of anaesthesia using an open breathing system with gauze and ether or chloroform. This might be carried out with the midwife, district nurse or even the patient's mother giving the anaesthetic via an open mask.[36] She was prepared to deliver at home patients that many GPs were happy to refer for hospital delivery. These might include forceps and breech deliveries, twins and elderly primipara. Dr Ockrim was determined to work in a co-operative fashion with the community midwives. She had been concerned about standards in some of the private nursing homes in the area and campaigned for them to improve or face closure. Study participants had good memories of their home deliveries as the following representative sample shows.

> The home would win all the time. I don't think that a hospital is the place to be when you need sympathy and understanding. . . . What I felt was—it was my decision to do what I was going to do at home.
>
> (INa)

> I booked my first baby at home, but complications arose. . . . The second baby was born at home. Dr Ockrim, herself, delivered him in the house. I preferred the home delivery. It was a different experience entirely. There was no comparison. The doctor was there the whole time and attended to you. In the hospital you were left quite a lot yourself to get on with it, but at home you had a student, a midwife and the doctor in attendance and everyone couldn't be nicer.
>
> (GT)

> Well, they say I'm old-fashioned, but I still preferred a house birth to a hospital birth. I believe in that. I think there is a closeness to the baby, plus if you have got any other family, you are there, and to me it is a happier feeling. My mother had six of us all in a room and kitchen [without an inside toilet].
>
> (RNc)

The nurse hadn't arrived, and I was having difficulty . . . and you said to my mother, 'You put that on—that mask and I'll leave my hands free for a minute' and you . . . got forceps and that was how you delivered her.

(INa)

I had taken pains in the morning and then the waters broke. I took my daughter to school, and I came down [to the surgery] to see you. You told me to go straight home—yes, I was in labour. It [the anaesthetic] was a thing you put over your face. My sister stood at the top of the bed and held this thing—it was tiny drops. [The nurse] stood at the side of the bed.

(GT)

Fitting in the time for home or nursing home deliveries and having a practice with fixed consulting times meant a constant juggling of commitments. Attending a difficult forceps birth might mean working through the night after a busy day in the practice. Patients were very appreciative of the input of doctor and midwife for home deliveries and especially when the delivery involved a considerable amount of time. While a product of its time, domiciliary obstetrics and the close involvement at every stage of the pregnancy proved to be a powerful force in the link between doctor and patient.

A final tribute to Dr Ockrim for her community obstetrics appeared in a letter to the editor of the (Glasgow) Herald on the 19th of September 2007, just one day after they had printed an obituary about her and her career. Headed 'Wonderful Woman', it read as follows:

Dear Sir,

Thank you for the tribute to Dr Ockrim Collins (September 19th). Dr Ockrim, as she was known, is a legend in our family, following my successful delivery in June 1962 in the family home in Drumoyne. My mother was a patient of Dr Ockrim's husband, Dr Collins, who was sensitive to the difficult labour and trauma of a sick baby my mother had suffered at the Southern General some years earlier and recommended his wife for a home delivery. Mum still recalls with affection the care she received from this wonderful lady. Ever outspoken, Dr Ockrim's only complaint about mum's preparation for, and co-operation during the birth was to voice dissatisfaction about the choice of my name as she had already delivered more than one Karen that week. Mum is now in her 77th year and shed more than just a few tears on reading the obituary.

Jim and Karen McQueen, 22 Nethercliffe Avenue, Netherlee, Glasgow

Health Visitors

Glasgow had a system of health visitors in pre-NHS days known as the Green Ladies, because of the colour of their uniform, who were employed by Glasgow Corporation. They offered advice on feeding, advocating breast feeding, hygienic food preparation and domestic cleanliness. However, Green Ladies were not always well received in homes. Some mothers resented what they considered to be an invasion of privacy, and health visitors were popularly believed to be quick to criticise. Sister French recalled the following:

> Yes, [the Green Ladies were held in awe]. It was fear, you know. It went through a street when she walked in. She was used in a wrong sense. She was the person who told them who kept their house and who didn't keep their house.
>
> It was your surgery I came to. . . . the Queen's Nurses wouldn't come to Abercrombie Street, so I had to get the Green Ladies and you didn't like them very much . . . so, when I went into labour—she was that intent on me gettin' an enema, that you came to the door before she had me ready and . . . she was that busy trying to get me to take an enema that you came to the door and you weren't very happy.
>
> (INa)

> Just the Green Ladies that came [for the delivery]. And the doctor. Of course, when they went out, I would get up and do things myself. . . . They [The Green Ladies] were in every morning. They cleaned me and they done the wee one. I remember the lady saying to me to try and take it easy.
>
> (CNk)

Nursing Homes and Hospital

Though there were maternity services available at the local Southern General Hospital, some mothers were encouraged, or even forced, to take the option of having their babies at overflow facilities at Lennox Castle Hospital at Lennoxtown at the foot of the Campsie Fells.[37] The hospital also housed a large facility for patients with learning disabilities, and the use of the maternity facilities, started on an emergency basis during World War II, lasted until the 1960s. Transport arrangements were difficult, so family visits were few.

> I was washing the floor and I took no' well and [my husband] ran and phoned the doctor and it was an ambulance that was sent, and the ambulance man took me first to the Southern General, but there was no vacancies, so he was told to go to Lennox Castle.
>
> (LD)

> The boys were delivered in Lennox Castle. I've no idea [why]. It was a terrible place to get to.
>
> (ZR)

> My husband and my sister-in-law came with me to Montrose St. That was the health centre place, and we got a van that took us to Lennox Castle. The families weren't allowed to go—just the patients in this van.
>
> (HNa)

For many years, as the number of genuine home deliveries decreased, Dr Ockrim did the bulk of her maternity work at the St Francis Nursing Home, a Catholic home near the practice, which had been opened in 1945 to uphold Catholic values related to termination of pregnancy and sterilisation. The Home supported mothers to have up to a dozen children delivered by section, and young unmarried mothers were given support to go through with their pregnancies.

While Dr Ockrim was greatly appreciative of the skills and care of the nuns at St Francis, not all the patients had the same attitude to childbirth in a nursing home with a strong Catholic ethos.

I don't think she was very happy there. I think—alright with [our first], it was—the second one. She was left, if I remember right. They were left on their own and they seemed to attend the Roman Catholics more. That was the impression I got. She didn't go back there.

(HT)

St Francis was very good, apart from all their ringing bells and that. Waking you up at all times in the morning. They didn't twist it, you know, [her] not being Catholic which was very good.

(VK)

I had gone to St Frances and was interviewed there, and they more or less booked my place to go and have the baby and when I went home and told my father—he didn't approve. He said, there is no grandchild of mine being born in a Catholic home. It was dreadful. My father was Highland, and I suppose that's [the reason].

(DR)

[Dr Ockrim] said, 'You can go to St Frances.' I said, 'I'm not a Catholic.' She said, 'That doesn't make any difference.' [It was] marvellous. They made no difference.

(IN)

The facilities at St Francis could not compare with the Southern General Hospital's new Maternity Unit, which opened around 1970. The presence of a GP unit within the new building meant that those general practitioners who wished to continue to offer full intra-partum care could still do so. At the same time, St Francis seemed to be struggling; midwife recruitment had been falling, and the costs of new equipment had become prohibitive. The GP unit at the Southern was equipped to deal with any emergencies so patients could have every level of care available in one place. It eventually closed because the GPs were becoming increasingly committed to core practice activities, and few younger doctors had the necessary experience.

The amenities were different. They were far superior, but I think the big, long ward was—you had more company. If you are going up and down the ward, you meet the whole ward as you are going back and forward to the toilet and so forth.

(IK)

I think it was yourself that delivered my second baby in the GP Unit at the Southern General. I preferred my own doctor to do the delivery because it was more personal. They were with you all through the pregnancy and I think it was nice to have them at the end of it. You felt comfortable.

(Elizabeth Whyteman)

After an initial period of enthusiasm, Dr Ockrim eventually found the time required at the hospital's GP unit too much of a conflict with practice requirements, and she withdrew from the service in 1980. She said the following:

I know myself, I stopped going because if I went in and to have a drip or something put up, there was never any staff, they were all too busy with the hospital side. . . . That was the reason I stopped.

One final recollection of a delivery at the Southern General was from a patient who had waited patiently in the corridor outside the ward all day before someone noticed that she had been there for a long time. The patient presumed that the staff were busy and that the ward was full so had been prepared to wait.

We phoned for the doctor, and he just phoned for the ambulance. I was in hospital at 11 o'clock that Wednesday morning and my mother came up at visiting in the afternoon and I was still sitting in this day room with poly bag and clothes. There was girls coming in and delivered and finished and away and I was still sitting there.

At midnight I got up with this bag of clothes in my hand. I'm walking down the corridor and by this time the place was dark. This Sister came up to me and said, 'What are you doing dear?' I said, 'I haven't got a bed'. She said, 'What do you mean you haven't got a bed?' I said, 'I've been here from 11 o'clock this morning and I haven't got a bed'. So, Sister got a hold of me. She was so shocked. They had obviously forgot about me and I wasnae creating any havoc, so that was ok.

(RNk)

Stillbirths, Maternal and Neonatal Deaths

The loss of a baby and, even more so, the death of a mother could have a profound effect on the family. One participant (DL) recalled, 'Yes, it was [a terrible tragedy]. She never got over them, my mother', and the family maintained a weekly visit to the cemetery for many years. Other participants remembered their own experience of stillbirth. One mother (DD) had experienced a fall, and she recalled, 'I had twin girls and lost them. That was a fall I had. I was full time'. Another mentioned the loss of a grandchild with spina bifida, who was 'dead on delivery'.

Other mothers were more fortunate, though only after being told that the foetus had died. One recalled that '[the baby] was born and there was nobody there. No nurse, no doctor. They discovered that he was still alive'. Another (EX) was told by the doctor that 'the baby was dead and unfortunately: they would have to section me'.

There was a delay in telling her the result of the section—she added, 'That was the only sad part about it, nobody had come and told me that the baby had lived'.

Changing Attitudes

Changes in society led to the beginnings of a male role in supporting their partners during the birth process. Special classes were organised for fathers so that they would have some familiarity with the delivery room procedures.

> He [my husband] was quite happy to be there. I think he found the first one— he wasn't actually in the room for the first one and he was in the room for the rest. I think I was quite glad. I don't think he would have been any less interested or caring if he hadn't been there, but I think it's quite good for him to be there because he might have felt a bit more sympathetic towards me later on! It was really great.
> I don't think he was any support at all, no. I think the pain is so excruciating you haven't really much time for anybody. I really felt I had to look after him because he was so upset at seeing me in pain that I had to pretend I wasn't in pain so that he would feel better. It would probably have been better if he hadn't been there. I wouldn't tell him that.
>
> (Linda McMahon)

> They are doing things all different. They're having their weans[38] and then getting engaged and then getting married. They do everything all stupid. I just leave them [my daughters] to it. As long as they don't come in and tell me they're pregnant, then I'm quite happy. They're no stupid lassies. All their pals—Agnes' pal was fifteen when she found out she was pregnant. She looks after the child herself. That's the way of the world now.
>
> (Elizabeth Whyteman)

In the past, many adopting parents did not tell the children they were bringing up that they had been adopted. One patient only discovered that she had been adopted when she received her pension book at the age of sixty:

> The reason I found out I didn't belong to them was when the pension book came through and they sent me a pension book. . . . I thought I had somebody else's pension book, so I ran up to the welfare place and asked to see somebody to hand the book back and apparently, I hadn't noticed [my name] at the end of it. She phoned up somewhere and they asked for my insurance number. They said that it was the proper book. I got a fright.
>
> (CNk)

One theme that emerges with many of the older patients is the prevalent level of sexual naivete. 'I knew what you had to do I suppose, but I can assure you that I was a virgin when I got married. . . . Even when I'm talking to you, I can feel my heart going' (FK). Some female patients were reticent to talk about intimate and sexual matters even with a woman doctor. There were examples of adolescents being terrified by the appearance of a first period, and the colloquial term for 'menstruation' was often described as an 'illness'. One participant (ZR) said the following:

> You didnae discuss these things. I was quite ignorant. It was mainly my grandparents that brought me up and [my grandmother] was very straight-laced and she wouldn't discuss anything like that.

The embarrassment about sexual matters extended to gynaecology investigations.

> Well, if you really want to know [why I've never attended the Well Woman Clinic] it's because I get the smear—I've never even had an internal. I've never . . . and I think I'm actually frightened.
>
> (DE)

These attitudes were not uncommon. A literature search identified studies that examine factors influencing women's participation in the cervical cytology screening programme, their psychological reaction to the receipt of an abnormal result and their experiences of colposcopy.[39] Reasons for non-participation include administrative failures, unavailability of a female screener, inconvenient clinic times, lack of awareness of the test's indications and benefits, consideration of oneself not to be at risk of developing cervical cancer and fear of embarrassment, pain or the detection of cancer. The fear of embarrassment or pain was mentioned frequently and occurs frequently in the literature.[40] Women of low socio-economic status or from ethnic minorities may be less likely to have been screened.[41] However, Dr Ockrim's well-kept book of the smear tests she performed and their results shows high levels of uptake with both groups from the start of her programme in 1966.[42]

Over the years, there were a few dramatic situations which were recalled by patients, staff and doctors. One of the most vivid occurred around 1950 and stood out in the memory of those present. The incident shows both a level of sexual naivety and desperation to find an answer to their problem. This concerned a couple who wanted information on the practicalities of sexual intercourse to the extent that they stripped off in front of Dr Ockrim. She recalled afterwards that she ran out of the room looking for help, an account remembered by one of the patients in the surgery at the time. It turned out that the male partners in the practice had been aware of the couple and their sexual difficulties and had merely suggested they consult Dr Ockrim together. Forty years later, she had still not resolved how the situation might have been handled better. VK recalled the following:

> It was two 'sort of retarded' people . . . but I did hear that they had wanted information on sex, and they wanted to do the act actually in the surgery, in your room—Of course, the 'natural thing' was to go and see your partner and then get them sorted out and get their clothes on.

In fact, the 'natural thing' as seen today would have been to elicit an understanding of their difficulties and appropriate counselling to see that their needs were addressed.

SEXUAL ABUSE

In the previous chapter, we encountered a patient that had accompanied her father to the surgery and had seen how Dr Ockrim had been able to confront her father about his drinking problem. However, there was a deeper and far more serious problem, unacknowledged at home. She had been experiencing physical and sexual abuse at the hands of her father, possibly even with the knowledge of her mother. She felt unable to confide in family members, but she did open up to a school friend. This was far from producing any resolution. The abuse had begun during the early 1970s when support services for victims of sexual abuse hardly existed and victims were reluctant to divulge what they had been experiencing.[43] The consequences of the abuse could be severe and long-lasting, often with a complete breakdown in family relationships.[44]

> Aye, I had a pal and her da' was da'en the same thing to her. Her da' was actually takin' photos of them having intercourse. It was one of thae cameras that just came oot. I told my pal that my da' took me to bed and she said, so does ma da'. We were all quite young.
>
> (DM)

The abuse continued for many years, and she was intimidated by the behaviour of her father who created false stories about her behaviour which ended up with her being held for a time in very inappropriate institutions.

> He made oot tae folk that I was sick in the heid. He made oot a lot of bad stories about me to people. It got to the stage the schoolboard took me to a Childrens' Panel and he wouldnae pay the £12 fine, so I was put into Lennox Castle Hospital.[45] I was there for two weeks and there was a doctor [who] said I shouldnae have been there.
>
> I know I'll never get over it, but I'll get on with my life and I tried to forgive my da' one day and he expected me to forgive him and then he started causing a riot and arguing and all that. He kept calling me a liar and 'he didnae dae anything'. So, he more or less didnae want tae be forgiven.
>
> Society is changing now. There should be more help and there should be better ways of dealing wi' it. Everybody's learning. Social workers are still learning. You've got to learn from your mistakes, so they're still learning. I reckon that they could learn better fae a person that has been abused. The person that's already had to deal wi' it.
>
> (DM)

CHILD HEALTH

Care of children is an important part of general practice, and the testimonies show how their children's illnesses were seen as well as the interaction of parents with the health care professionals. Iain Hutchison notes that it was not until the 1986 edition of Rosa Sacharin's *Principles of Paediatric Nursing* that nurses were recommended to obtain a rapport with the parents and to understand the psychology of their young charges.[46] One patient remembered the following:

> I remember when you go to Belvedere, [with an infectious disease] your parents weren't tae get in then. When you went in there was a waiting room [for parents to see their children] and a long wall with windows along the top.
>
> (LI)

For Dr Ockrim, this relationship was important from the start. She was determined to help parents see their offspring develop to their full potential. The wall of her consulting room was filled with pictures that her child patients, or their parents, had given her over the more than forty years of her practice. She recalled the following:

> Children used to bring in the photographs that they got taken at school and of course, when they came in, they liked to see their pictures on the wall, so I had quite a collection of children's photographs.

As Lawrence Weaver has pointed out, the history of child health in Western countries has seen the emergence of the baby as an individual out of the darkness of early death, uncertain survival, parental resignation and public indifference.[47] By the end of the nineteenth century, high rates of infant mortality had become a subject of social and political concern and began to attract medical interest. Glasgow's history of social deprivation and inequalities in health care was perhaps more obviously visible in the field of paediatrics. It would take some time from the inauguration of the National Health Service for the much-needed improvements to child health to take effect.

The history of Glasgow's Royal Hospital for Sick Children gives ample evidence of the dirt-poor hygiene and unwashed clothing seen on admission even in the first years of the NHS.[48] Hutchison described the aura of mystique, and autocratic practices, by specialist hospital paediatrics in these first years of the National Health Service, amply confirmed by extensive interviews with former staff.[49] While parents were useful in obtaining the history of their children, consultants generally felt that families shouldn't have to worry about what was wrong. The days of understanding the psychology of young children remained firmly in the future.[50]

Communication Issues

Study participants recalled which emphasised the difficulty of parent and hospital staff communication in the early days. In this memory, the parents eventually made the decision to take the child home, where, fortunately, the symptoms just disappeared.

> I think he was a year and four months. He had just started to toddle—You know how they toddle about. This morning I got him up and he couldn't

stand. His legs just kept going away from him and I tried to get him to stand up, but no. . . . He got an ambulance and took him to the Southern and they kept him in there for 10 days and they didnae discover what had brought that on. This day I'd been down—the wee soul—he was tied to the end of the cot.

(INa)

Given the mother's anxiety, the father brought the child home where he made a rapid recovery. Another parent recalled that he and his wife 'weren't all that pleased with the hospital there'. The staff were described as 'too domineering' and 'as far as the children were concerned and . . . they weren't nice to the kids at all'. He didn't take the matter up with the staff as that would have 'upset us more' (VK). A mother, with experience of a handicapped child described the attitude of the obstetrician as follows:

all wrong—he would examine you—no conversation and look doon on you and back oot the door again.' Maybe it was just me, I don't know.

(LH)

The General Medical Council recommended in 1967, that 'the growing child should be studied in his family setting and in association with members of the domiciliary services'.[51] Statutory child welfare clinics had been well established by the end of World War II with a decline in infant mortality and the greater reliability of health visitors attending newborns following the Notification of Birth Act.[52] Although hospital paediatric experience was part of the preparation for general practice, an article in the *Journal of the Royal College of General Practitioners*, at the time of the interviews, asked if paediatrics was safe in general practitioners' hands.[53] It commented that few older doctors had qualifications and experience in paediatrics, and the doctors studied differed widely in their management of hypothetical clinical problems, possibly owing to this lack of training.

One participant's memory was of two years spent in hospital after an unspecified event when she was nine years old. She has no knowledge of a diagnosis, received no treatment and was eventually discharged.

I got a fright, during the black out in 1939. On the Saturday he [Dr George] came to the house and I was in Yorkhill Sick Children's Hospital on the Sunday. I was in Yorkhill Hospital for a year and Stobhill Hospital and then a year in Drumchapel. [No treatment], just complete rest. I enjoyed it, believe it or not, I really enjoyed it.

(TNr)

One mother changed to the practice because of a lack of understanding of her emotional needs after experiencing a cot death.[54] Having explained how the practice was able to support her at a vulnerable time, Linda McMahon described the cot death and the impact it had on her and her family and why she changed to a different doctor. She made it clear that patient support is more than just the prescription of Valium.

It was a cot death. I just felt the [previous] GP's attitude was very rigid. I always felt he made all the moves, and he dictated the terms on which our relationship was going to be based and it was very much a doctor-patient relationship, in the old-fashioned sense, rather than being a person-to-person relationship. I never felt I got to know him at all on friendly terms. He came up and left a lot of Valium and didn't come back again. We could have done with more support.

On moving to the practice, she recalled that 'as a practice, the doctors I go to are very supportive and you form a relationship with them which I never really did [before]'.

A more distant memory concerned tonsillectomy, at one time one of the most widely practised surgical procedures, though with doubtful benefit in most cases.[55] Indeed, tonsillectomy had been such a popular procedure that the stories of the operation being carried out on the kitchen table were part of the legend of general practice.[56] The following is a patient recollection of the removal of tonsils and adenoids, before WWII, which mentions the weakness of the clinical base for surgery and the traumatic way in which the procedure was carried out.

Eventually she [my mother] got it into her head that I needed my tonsils cut. Tonsil cutting was a fashion then. You never hear much of it now. . . . I had no sore throat or anything at the time. I think [the doctor] was like me and she convinced him, and I think he did it for a quiet life too. He said, 'Ok, I'll get his tonsils out.' . . . The experience when I did get them cut was quite traumatic. There was a whole lot of little children, and we were all herded along to the operating theatre, and I had one of the babies to carry and we sat outside the door of the operating theatre and the children went in one by one and the terrible thing was that they came out facing us. We were sitting there on a form[57] and the children came out carried by a nurse and there was blood all over their face and running down their fronts and this had a terrible effect on us.

(ZN)

Yes. It was obvious to me that there should have been facilities for his mother to stay with him. I understand they do that now. Strangely enough, in primitive places, when I worked in Persia [in the 1930s] and these kinds of places, the hospital was very crude, but the family was along there when a person went in.

(ZN)

Of course, in more recent years, facilities are provided for parents to be in hospital with their children. A mother whose son was undergoing cardiac surgery recalled how she welcomed the opportunity to be able to stay in hospital with her children:

Oh yes . . . I don't think I could have got through it otherwise . . . because before his operation, obviously the medical students want to learn all about the different heart complaints, and he was being taken away all the time and

I was pleased that I could be with him when there was all these strangers examining him.

(KNk)

In an emergency situation, it can be difficult to make the right decision, and sometimes, the advice from professionals can be challenging even if later they seem to have made sense.

It just happened one day, I was to go and feed him and bath him and when I walked into the ward, I could see doctors and nurses running everywhere, I never thought for a minute that they were at my son. He [the doctor] came in and said, 'I don't think your son is gonnae make it, he's just taken another attack and he's in a coma'. I was stunned. I thought, I'm just here myself and totally shocked. I said, 'What dae I do?' He said, 'My advice to you is, I don't want you to go in'.

I thought no. I didnae like it. Looking back, he was obviously right. Looking back, he was saying it for my benefit as well as my husband, but you don't really think at that point.

(LH)

The interviews were conducted around the time that the whooping cough vaccine was being questioned for safety and side effects. Fortunately, when many children in the practice had what parents thought was a whooping cough, it turned out to be a much milder infection rather than one caused by *Bordetella pertussis*. The only reference to whooping cough concerned the vaccination dilemma:

They've all had their injections except for the whooping cough. Well at the time when our first was due her whooping cough there was a scare about the injection, maybe causing brain damage and my father-in-law had been epileptic and the danger of the inoculation seemed worse than the actual illness itself.... No, fortunately [none of them had whooping cough] or I would have felt dreadful for not having them inoculated.

(Linda McMahon)

Meningitis

Amongst acute infections, the most feared by parents has been meningitis, as its effects in young children can be devastating. Difficult to diagnose in its early stages, the condition can be life-threatening because of the inflammation's proximity to the brain and spinal cord. The condition is classified as a medical emergency, and immediate hospitalisation is essential. Because of the difficulty with diagnosis, communication problems between parents that understood the behaviour of their children and hospital doctors was vividly described.

I was shattered, I couldn't believe it. We kept insisting that there was something wrong. Because it was our first baby, they just seemed to think they knew better, and it wasn't till the third time that they actually saw him taking a fit. Then they started to believe that there was something seriously wrong with him.

(AK)

Just a couple of years ago I had [fostered] a wee boy and when he got up on the Saturday morning he got up and his neck was sore, and his throat was sore, and I thought—that's meningitis. I phoned the surgery right away and the doctor came out and he said, 'Oh there's nothing wrong with him. He's kidding you on, tell him to get up and play.' All that morning I kept watching the wee fella and he was staggering, as though he was drunk. I thought, no, there's definately something. So, I phoned stand-by and told them about it, and they said, 'Right, we'll back you up. We'll send you a taxi and take him right over to Yorkhill.' So, I took him over there, and he got a lumbar puncture done and it was meningitis. So of course, the next time I saw the doctor I told him what I thought of him. He said, 'I'm really sorry but I really did think he was kidding on.' I said, 'I told you he wasn't. . . . He's not a wee boy that kids on. He's a wee boy that's always lively.' I said, 'You should have listened to me when you came into my house. I don't normally make mistakes when it comes to kids.'

(HNi)

In this next memory, we have a child who had a history of febrile convulsions that had frequent encounters with paediatric hospital staff. When he develops meningitis, there is a reluctance of the hospital staff to make the diagnosis. The father recalled the following:

The second time we saw the child doctor, yes and it was ok . . . about taking the wee fits, but they always say—'a mother's instinct'. The next day, I came home from work, and I saw [him] taking one of the fits. That was the first time I saw him. It was as if he was holding his breath and I took him straight to the Southern and this time they took us up to the children's ward. The doctor saw him taking a fit and the next thing he was called for a lumbar puncture. It was meningitis he had, and he was transferred to Yorkhill. The first time we went to see him in intensive care he had probes in his head and tubes. We were told the next twenty-four hours were crucial, but he managed to pull through that.

(AK)

[Dr Ockrim] phoned an ambulance and I said, 'What's wrong with her?' No answer. The ambulance came and I went to the hospital with [an older daughter]. They took her away. I think it was Ruchill. They took her away and the Sister came and took me into a room, and she said, 'I'm afraid your daughter has got meningitis'. I burst into tears. . . . I saw the doctor in the hospital, and I said, 'It couldn't have been meningitis then'. He said, 'Yes, I'm afraid it was. Only for your doctors quick thinking' he said, 'Only very few doctors can diagnose that.' I had to thank Dr Ockrim for that.

(IH)

Well, when I was a year old [in 1927]—I was told [later] I had meningitis. [I was] in Ruchill [Hospital] for a long, long time. The report line was out for me, and my father got the minister in Admiral Street Church to call to the hospital. He said a prayer. One of the people in the hospital suggested to my mother there was a chance, but she would need to sign some document and they explained to her what they were going to do. It was a chance, you know. They said they were thinking if they cut part of the toe that the disease would—this was before modern medicine. . . . So, my mother signed the paper anyway. She suggested my ear because the hair would cover it. It was decided that it didnae matter what part—the disease would come through this way. I got home a fortnight after that. It is [an 'old wives' tale'], but in saying that, I have it and other people have it. There's something to it.

(DD)

Patient Support Groups

Both the mother who had experienced the cot death of a child and the mother of a child with congenital heart disease attended support groups. Different parents have different expectations of such groups, but they are widely acknowledged to be helpful in providing information and emotional support. The first mother benefitted both from the counselling and information provided and was prepared to speak to other parents; the second acknowledged the support she had received from counsellors but was much more ambivalent in speaking to other parents and becoming involved in group discussions. These thoughtful testimonies describe the benefits and some drawbacks of patient groups.

I've been attending an Association for Children with Heart Disorders and a lot of people don't always want to know things that I wanted to know. A lot of people don't want to know the details of what's going to happen to their child. I do, but I can't tell someone else that they must ask questions and know all the details if they don't want to know them. They have to want to know that themselves. That's when I think it's difficult for me to tell someone what they should do.

I got as much support as I asked for in the form of questions. I asked a lot of questions. I probably needed a wee bit more support and I actually phoned up a charity and I asked if they had any literature regarding children's heart operations, and she just said no, she didn't have anything like that at all. I would have liked to have had literature to read. I don't know that I was ready for the Association for Children with Heart Disorders, before [the] operation. I think I was too nervous about what the future would hold, to discuss it just with strangers. I needed literature and there wasn't any at that time. I think they have to ask the questions still. I don't think a doctor will say, this might happen or that might happen. You have to ask questions.

Well, I suppose when I was in hospital, I did find out, through the system, that there was such an Association, and I went and contacted them. To be honest I have mixed feelings. When you are admitted you see one person after another, and your head is spinning. I really don't know if that's the right time to see parents. You don't know what's ahead of you and you are worried, and you see so many people. There was a social worker in the hospital and before [the] operation I went along to a meeting. . . . Two of the other mothers that were there, their children had had their operations the week before. Those mothers were quite relaxed and ready to ask questions, but I wasn't. I had to make sure he got through the operation first. The social worker said to me at the end, 'Well do you feel better now?' I said, 'No I don't, nothing could make me feel good at this stage'. So, I think maybe the time is after the surgery, when you're more prepared.

(KNk)

Well, the Cot Death Trust at Yorkhill[58]—we went to see them, but that was completely of our own suggestion. They were wonderful. I can't praise them enough; they were just wonderful. Just the way they talked to you, the way they treated you. They sent a health visitor to come and see us and kept in touch. To know that it happened to other people. No, there weren't very many people locally who had [a similar experience] and I didn't really want to [speak to other parents] at the time. I can't really remember why now. I think I felt my own experience was so intensely personal that no-one else could possibly understand what it was. Now I think I'm wrong, I think they probably could have, but at the time I didn't. [Self-help groups are good] for people who prefer a communal experience rather than getting over things by an effort of your will, then they provide a great deal of support. I don't know if I would like that.

(Linda McMahon)

Fostering

Fostering children was a topic mentioned a few times by different interviewees. The provision of foster care has been a difficult area for local authorities to monitor, as they try to ensure that foster parents provide the 'nurture and unconditional love (that) are fundamental to caring for damaged and vulnerable children'.[59] Intervening with the most vulnerable children in their very early months and years of life can reap large rewards for that child, the family and the whole of society. At-risk children have major health and lifespan risks: increased risk of mental health problems, such as conduct disorders, depression and suicide, but also physical illness. Children with an early persistent conduct disorder go on, as adults, to commit half of all crime.

General practitioners are involved during the fostering process, as medical assessments have to be carried out regularly, and they provide the care for the fostered child while they are with the family looking after the child. There were problems noted in securing safe, nurturing permanent placements for abused and neglected children, many of whom moved to and fro between maltreating birth families and temporary foster placements. Glasgow fostering primarily involves social services, whereby social workers assess the family and help to engage them with support and clinical services.

One of those interviewed was a highly skilled foster mother, caring in the short term for children that had social and health issues, while bringing up her own family. The following interviews mainly show fostering within the framework of the Social Work Department, but the last two show how care can be arranged for children when a surviving parent can no longer cope and even the very informal arrangements by a Catholic priest to place an orphaned illegitimate child with a family that had just suffered the death of a baby during World War I.

The children that we get in are actually on a 'place of safety order', with it being a crisis situation they're coming in, and the parents know that if they keep that child then they will get into trouble with the police. . . . When people come in here to see their children, I don't make them feel—'Oh you shouldnae have done that, it's all your fault this child's here'. I try to talk to them as I would talk to any person and try not to discriminate against them. I find that way that they'll feel relaxed, and they'll talk to you about what's happened and why it's happened. I've got to say to them, 'Well look, I know you've told me this, but I've got to tell the social worker, or I will get into bother'. They'll say, 'That's ok, but do you mind if I try and tell her before you'.

The fostering situation could be a lot better. You could put a lot more support from the social workers than you do get.

(HNi)

Yes, my brother-in-law was left with the three kids and then he couldn't cope and that's when he started to drink. . . . So, the social worker came up and seen me. They came up to see me and I told them I had been helping with the kids. I'd more or less took them up here because o' him drinking. He says, 'If you want, I can put you on to fostering, if your brother's agreeable, and you'll get money to help you out tae keep them'. So, it all sort of stemmed from that and I'm their foster parent right up tae [she] left school there and started work.

(BC)

This big Irish priest kept saying to my mother, 'You know, if you take that child and bring it up, you're not losing out because you've just lost a child and God will put all the graces upon you and I can assure you that your husband will come back safe and sound [from World War I]'.

(LM)

This chapter recounts stories of participants' memories as they recalled encounters with general practitioners and hospital doctors and nurses. While medical staff usually know what the patient is describing in health terms, in many of these stories, things go wrong because symptoms are not believed, and when the facts emerge, as DR recalled, 'the surgeon just shrugged'. These memories feature what in many ways was the core of the oral history study: child-care, health issues, stigma and, above all, Dr Ockrim and her practice of obstetrics. In the three decades since these interviews took place, there has been a more open attitude to patient concerns, but GP deliveries are a thing of the past, and 'you still have to ask questions'.

NOTES

1 Boaking: Retching.
2 It is doubtful that the most junior doctor would have turned away a patient more than once without conferring with someone more senior. Perhaps there were others who should have been embarrassed, too.
3 Prior to hospital management reorganisation, the hospital was essentially run by the medical superintendent and the matron.
4 Period.
5 www.gla.ac.uk/schools/medicine/mus/ourfacilities/. history/20thcentury/1948-2018/nephrology/ (accessed 21 March 2021).
6 On a domiciliary visit.
7 Normally carried out for complete rectal prolapse. Harold Ellis, Professor of Surgery in the University of London, one of the most outstanding surgeons of his generation, started using the technique in 1961. All travel and accommodation costs for the patient and her mother were covered by the NHS.
8 Henry Tankel (1926–2010) was a consultant general surgeon at the Southern General Hospital in an era where the Surgical Department performed operations, such as prostate and thyroid surgery, now normally carried out by specialist surgeons. He had a distinguished role in medical politics and was a leading figure in Scotland's Jewish community.
9 Mr D. A. Peebles-Brown, Consultant Surgeon at the Western Infirmary, Glasgow, included this case in his paper: P. V. Walsh, D. A. Peebles-Brown, and G. Watkinson, Colectomy for Slow Transit Constipation, *Annals of the Royal College of Surgeons of England*, 69 (2), 1987, pp. 71–75. The study described the results in twenty-one patients, of whom only twelve responded fully to the surgery and two required an ileostomy.
10 R. Pugsley and Jenney Pardoe, The Specialist Contribution to the Care of the Terminally Ill Patient: Support or Substitution? *Journal of the Royal College of General Practitioners*, 36, 1986, pp. 347–348.
11 This is reminiscent of the poem of Emily Dickinson: (verse 1263) 'Tell all the truth but tell it slant' *The Poems of Emily Dickinson: Reading Edition* (Cambridge and London, The Belknap Press of Harvard University Press, 1998).
12 Irvine Loudon and Mark Drury, Clinical Care in General Practice, in Irvine Loudon, John Horder, and Charles Webster, *General Practice under the National Health Service 1948–1997* (Clarendon Press, London, 1998), p. 120.
13 Catherine Meredith, Paul Symonds, Lorraine Webster, Douglas Lamont, Elspeth Pyper, Charles R. Gillis, and Lesley Fallowfield, Information Needs of Cancer Patients in West Scotland: Cross Sectional Survey of 'Patients' Views, *British Medical Journal*, 313, 1996, p. 724. The study interviewed cancer patients who were selected by age, sex, socio-economic status and tumour site to be representative of cancer patients in the West of Scotland.
14 See, for example, the following Glasgow-based study: A. Montazeri, D. J. Hole, R. Milroy, et al., Does Knowledge of Cancer Diagnosis Affect Quality of Life? A Methodological Challenge, *BMC Cancer*, 4 (21), 2004. https://doi.org/10.1186/1471-2407-4-21.
15 Ali Montazeri, Robert Milroy, David Hole, James McEwen, and Charles R. Gillis, Anxiety and Depression in Patients with Lung Cancer Before and After Diagnosis: Findings from a Population in Glasgow, Scotland, *Journal of Epidemiology and Community Health*, 52, 1998, pp. 203–204.

16 R. Pugsley and Jenney Pardoe, The Specialist Contribution, pp. 347–348.
17 Ali Montazeri et al., ibid: see also Vera Carstairs and Russell Morris, *Deprivation and Health in Scotland* (Aberdeen University Press, Aberdeen, 1991), pp. 148–152.
18 A. Gregor, C. S. Thomson, D. H. Brewster, P. L. Stroner, J. Davidson, R. Fergusson, and R. Milroy, Management and Survival of Patients with Lung Cancer in Scotland Diagnosed in 1995: Results of a National Population-Based Study, *Scottish Cancer Trials Lung Group and the Scottish Cancer Therapy Network*. https://thorax.bmj.com/content/56/3/212.full (accessed 25 October 2020); see also Philip McLoone and F. A. Boddy, Deprivation and Mortality in Scotland, 1981 and 1991, *British Medical Journal*, 309, 1995, p. 1465, where it indicates that lung cancer mortality was falling faster in more affluent areas.
19 Margaret Kindlen, Hospice Home Care Services: A Scottish Perspective, *Palliative Medicine*, 2, 1988, pp. 115–121.
20 Sir Robert Wright DSO OBE (1915–1981) was the president of the General Medical Council of Great Britain, former president of the Royal College of Physicians and Surgeons of Glasgow, and surgeon-in-charge at the Southern General Hospital from 1953.
21 V. A. Hundley, F. M. Cruickshank, G. D. Lang, et al., Midwife Managed Delivery Unit: A Randomised Controlled Comparison with Consultant Led Care, *British Medical Journal*, 309, 1994, p. 1400. However, other studies have emphasised the safety of GP deliveries; see Marjorie Tew, Place of Birth and Perinatal Mortality, *Journal of the Royal College of General Practitioners*, 35 (277), 1985, pp. 390–394; M. Tew, The Case against Hospital Deliveries: The Statistical Evidence, in S. Kitzinger and J. A. Davies, editors, *The Place of Birth* (Oxford University Press, Oxford, 1978), pp. 55–65; M. Klein, I. Lloyd, C. Redman, et al., A Comparison of Low-Risk Women Booked for Delivery in Two Systems of Care: Shared Care (Consultant) and Integrated General Practice Unit, *British Journal of Obstetrics and Gynaecology*, 90, 1983, pp. 118–128.
22 NCT Policy Briefing: Choice of Place of Birth, November 2011, chrome-extension://efaidnbmnnnibpcajpcglclefindmkaj/viewer. html?pdfurl=https%3A%2F%2Fwww.nct.org.uk%2Fsites%2Fdefault%2Ffiles %2Frelated_documents%2FChoice%2520of%2520place%2520of%2520birth. pdf&clen=247929&chunk=true (accessed 24 April 2022).
23 Scudded: Slapped or smacked (Scots).
24 Sir John Peel (1904–2005) was a president of both the Royal College of Obstetricians and Gynaecologists, and the British Medical Association.
25 *Report of the Royal College of Obstetricians and Gynaecologists*, 1982, p. 9.
26 M. J. V. Bull, The General Practitioner Accoucheur in the 1980s, p. 367.
27 *The Role of General Practice in Maternity Care*, Occasional Paper 72, Royal College of General Practitioners, November 1995.
28 Rona Campbell and Alison Macfarlane, Debate on the Place of Birth, in Lindsay Reid, editor, *Midwifery: Freedom to Practise? An International Exploration of Midwifery Practice* (Churchill Livingstone, Edinburgh), pp. 217–233.
29 Lindsay Reid, *Midwifery in Scotland—A History* (Scottish History Press, Erskine, 2011), p. 24.
30 Howdies were still working in Glasgow as late as 1947. See Lindsay Reid, *Midwifery in Scotland*, p. 24.
31 Lindsay Reid, *Scottish Midwives: Twentieth-Century Voices* (Black Devon Books, Dunfermline, 2000). One of the midwives interviewed was Anne

Chapman, who had been working at Rottenrow while Dr Ockrim was a medical student. She recalled many instances of childbirth, in early 1940s, in seriously primitive circumstances of a kind never experienced in these interviews. She described deliveries in the basement area of tenement buildings with trodden earth floors, where squatters would move in and erect sacking partitions for privacy (p. 64).

32 Lindsay Reid, *Midwifery in Scotland*, p. 61.

33 Ibid., p. 62. The high levels of maternal mortality and the measures needed to deal with them were highlighted in two reports during the 1930s: Douglas and McKinley Report (1935) and the Cathcart Report (1936).

34 Lindsay Reid, Normal Birth in Scotland: The Effects of Policy, Geography and Culture, in Lindsay Reid, editor, *Midwifery: Freedom to Practise? An International Exploration of Midwifery Practice* (Churchill Livingstone, Edinburgh, 2007), pp. 240–260.

35 See, for example, Sarah Robinson, Maintaining the Independence of the Midwifery Profession: A Continuing Struggle, in Jo Garcia, Robert Kilpatrick, and Martin Richards, editors, *The Politics of Maternity Care: Services for Childbearing Women in Twentieth-Century Britain* (Clarendon Press, Oxford, 1990), pp. 71–86; Richard Johnstone, Mary Newburn, and Alison Macfarlane, Has the Medicalisation of Childbirth Gone Too Far? *British Medical Journal*, 324, 2002, pp. 892–895.

36 Comments on Dr Ockrim in interview with Margaret French.

37 Anne Bayne gives her account of working as midwife at Lennox Castle with patients from the poorer neighbourhoods of Glasgow in Lindsay Reid, *Scottish Midwives*, pp. 93–95.

38 Wean: Young child (Scots).

39 F. Fylan, Screening for Cervical Cancer: A Review of 'Women's Attitudes, Knowledge, and Behaviour, *British Journal of General Practice*, 48 (433), 1998, pp. 1509–1514.

40 H. Campbell, S. MacDonald, and M. McKiernan, Promotion of Cervical Screening Uptake by Health Visitor Follow-Up of Women Who Repeatedly Failed to Attend, *Journal of Public Health Medicine*, 18, 1996, pp. 94–97; R. K. Peters, B. Moraye, M. S. Bear, and D. Thomas, Barriers for Screening Cancers of the Cervix, *Preventive Medicine*, 18, 1989, pp. 133–146; A. K. Elkind, D. Haran, A. Eardley, and B. Spencer, Computer-Managed Cervical Cytology Screening: A Pilot Study of Non-Attenders, *Public Health*, 101, 1987, pp. 253–266.

41 B. R. McAvoy and R. Raza, Can Health Education Increase Uptake of Cervical Smear Testing among Asian Women? *BMJ*, 302, 1991, pp. 833–836.

42 Dr Hetty Ockrim, Cervical Cytology Ledger, in possession of the author.

43 The Women's Support Project only began in the city's East End in 1983. See Patricia Bell and Jan Macleod, Bridging the Gap: Feminist Development Work in Glasgow, *Feminist Review*, 28 (1), 1988, pp. 136–143.

44 Anne E. Stern, Deborah Lynch, R. Kim Oates, Brian I. 'O'Toole, and George Cooney, Self Esteem, Depression, Behaviour and Family Functioning in Sexually Abused Children, *Journal of Child Psychology and Psychiatry*, 36 (6), 1995, pp. 1077–1089.

45 Hospital catering for children with learning disabilities.

46 Iain Hutchison, Malcolm Nicolson, and Lawrence Weaver, *Child Health in Scotland: A History of Glasgow's Royal Hospital for Sick Children* (Scottish History Press, Erskine, 2016), p. 212.

47 L. Weaver, Focussing the Medical Gaze on the Newborn Baby, *Lancet*, 368, 2006, pp. 1059–1060.

48 Iain Hutchison, Malcolm Nicolson, and Lawrence Weaver, *Child Health in Scotland: A History of Glasgow's Royal Hospital for Sick Children* (Scottish History Press, Erskine, 2016), pp. 137–138.

49 Ibid., p. 142.

50 Ibid., p. 212.

51 General Medical Council, *Recommendations as to Basic Medical Education* (GMC, London, 1967).

52 Lawrence T. Weaver, In the Balance: Weighing Babies and the Birth of the Infant Welfare Clinic, *Bulletin of the History of Medicine*, 84, 2010, pp. 30–57.

53 Geoffrey N. Marsh, Daphne Russell, and Ian T. Russell, Is Paediatrics Safe in General 'Practitioners' Hands? A Study in the North of England, *Journal of the Royal College of General Practitioners*, 39, 1989, pp. 138–141.

54 The participant admitted to becoming 'over-protective'. For a summary of the necessary family support after a cot death see R. Walker, Cot Deaths: The Aftermath, *Journal of the Royal College of General Practitioners*, 35 (273), 1985, pp. 194–196: B. H. Zebal and S. F. Woolsey, SIDS and the Family: The Pediatrician's Role, *Pediatric Annals*, 13, 1984, pp. 237–261.

55 There were over 78,000 tonsillectomies carried out in England during 1994 and 1995, but that benefit could only be shown in patient who met very strict clinical criteria; see Tom Marshall, A Review of Tonsillectomy for Recurrent Throat Infections, *British Journal of General Practice*, 48, 1998, pp. 1331–1335.

56 A. F. Wright asked, in an editorial titled 'All Our Tomorrows', in *British Journal of General Practice*, 1998, pp. 1375–1376, looking back at conditions in general practice in the 1940s, Will their recollection be of tonsillectomy on the kitchen table with the sweet smell of ether? Kitchen table tonsillectomies took place further afield, too. Bruce Halliday, working in general practice in Canada, recalled in an editorial: *Services then were partially aimed to keep health care costs to a minimum, because patients were largely responsible for payment. For example, we did tonsillectomies and adenoidectomies at patients' homes on the kitchen table, with Dr Taylor doing the surgery and me doing the anaesthesia* (Bruce Halliday, Editorial, *Canadian Family Physician/Le Médecin de famille Canadien*, 50, June/Juin 2004, pp. 845–847). This was also true of Australia: T. C. K. Brown, From Kitchen Table to Operating Theatre, *Pediatric Anesthesia*, 24, 2014, pp. 528–530.

57 Form: Bench (Scots).

58 The Scottish Cot Death Trust was founded in 1985 to provide support for bereaved families and educate the public and professionals about sudden unexpected death in infants (SUDI).

59 Kirstie Maclean, Fostering and Adoption in Scotland: 1980–2010, *Adoption and Fostering*, 34 (3), 2010, pp. 21–25; Jo Dixon and Mike Stein, *A Study of Throughcare and Aftercare Services in Scotland. 'Scotland's Children: Children (Scotland) Act 1995, Research Findings No. 3* (Scottish Executive Education Department, Edinburgh).

7

Discussion and Conclusion

Memory and history confront each other across the tape recorder.[1]

The interviewees emphasised the importance of the presence of a caring physician, especially one that they had seen through their life experiences, and those of their extended families, and had come to trust implicitly. Timely access to their doctor was important, and there was considerable suspicion of the proposed appointments system which they feared would create a barrier between them and their GP. The study brought many aspects of social history to the fore. The tenement slums had engendered a sense of togetherness which had now been lost.

Dr Ockrim always reckoned that her obstetric work was a key component of general practice. Most mothers agreed, while understanding that the medicalisation of childbirth could not be reversed. Vivid memories of illnesses showed how these events came to be understood in terms that could be easily understood. The chapter on addictions reveals the struggle with alcohol and latterly with drugs, which destroyed the lives of addicts and split families apart. Like the ghost of times past was the memory of the pre-NHS days where patients struggled to pay for a consultation or a house call, or had to accept humiliation from the parish system and the poorhouse.

A presence in these interviews was Dr Ockrim herself. In the interviews, she allowed the participants to express their memories in their own way, and her own feelings were very rarely expressed. Recalled with affection by many of her former patients, she was credited by some with the intervention that saved them or their children from certain death. Her personality enabled female patients to have an enhanced sense of themselves and gave many the support and encouragement to follow what they saw as their destiny. These images were enhanced by the 'Letters to No-One' which encapsulated the hopes and fears of a busy city general practitioner looking to an uncertain future at retirement.

Oral history provides a window into how individuals understand and interpret their lives. Testimonies from oral histories are, by their nature, very subjective. Consequently, many researchers have noted that, just as in other types of evidence, the material recorded in oral history interviews will display varying levels of accuracy, requiring researchers to take care in examining their sources. Memories may even clash with the prior understandings of the researcher. Paul Thompson points to the paradox at the heart of oral history:

DOI: 10.1201/9781003369301-7

Any historical work suffers the inevitable disadvantage of having to work from the real cases available rather than created from specially created experiments.[2]

We have noted how Alessandro Portelli considered that oral history adds meaning and that 'wrong' statements are still psychologically 'true'.[3] Mark Roseman commented on Holocaust survivors showing minor inaccuracies in testimony, which could be related to the trauma of the event.[4] Lawrence Langer also confirmed that 'the troubled interaction between past and present achieves a gravity that surpasses the concern with accuracy'.[5]

This study is pioneering, as the product of the interview encounter by a general practitioner with her former patients, providing their unmediated views. At the same time, it relies on methods of recording and interpretation developed during the development of oral history practices. An oral history of local general practice was conducted in nearby Paisley through interviews with retired and practising GPs, providing their account of the views of their patients and showing a positive interaction between practice doctors and those in the hospital.[6]

The Paisley study, of Smith and Nicolson, relied for interpretation on the works of Schrager, Bakhtin and Portelli. Schrager attempted to identify elements in individual narratives that symbolise larger trends and social understandings, being particularly interested in the complexity of positions adopted within individual oral histories.[7] Bakhtin, like Schrager, sees many 'voices' in the diversity of individual accounts, which contributes to making oral history 'social'.[8] These individual testimonies create a 'form of dialogue' between the interviewees, and the social context is, therefore, crucial to understanding.

Besides the meaning that oral history provides, which has already been referred to, Portelli points out that what makes oral history different is the following:

1. The unique and precious element which oral sources force upon the historian and which no other sources possess in equal measure is the speaker's subjectivity: and therefore, if the research is broad and articulated enough, a cross-section of the subjectivity of a social group or class.[9]
2. The credibility of oral sources is a different credibility. The importance of oral testimony may often lie not in its adherence to facts but rather in its divergence from them, where imagination, symbolism, desire break in. Therefore, there are no 'false' oral sources.[10]
3. A strange by-product of this prejudice (against oral history) is the insistence that oral sources are distant from events and, therefore, undergo distortions deriving from faulty memory—In fact, historians have often used written sources which were written long after the actual events.

Trevor Lummis argued that social interpretation, as Samuel Schrager had done, became the standard understanding of oral history. Paul Thompson described interpretation as 'the heart of the matter', asking how we relate the evidence we have found to 'wider patterns and theories of history'.[11] He reminds us that 'the tension which the oral historian feels is that of the mainspring: between history and real life'[12] and considers that 'the oral evidence is treated as a quarry from which to construct an argument',[13] noting that interviews can give us 'information as valid as that obtainable from any other human source'.[14]

While one would not normally seek to use oral history on its own to build a standard history of past events, it is also true that, as Alistair Thomson writes, 'oral history is essential evidence for analysis of between past and present, and between memory and mythology'.[15] Thomson described how memories are composed to make sense of our past and present; he notes this:

> We remake or repress memories of experiences which are still painful or 'unsafe' because . . . their inherent traumas or tensions have never been resolved.

Richard Smith reminds that oral sources are themselves already analytic documents structured with complex codes and achieved meanings.[16] Lynn Abrams tells us that interpretation and meaning are important parts of the understanding of the interview and that the narrative and its interpretation belong together:

> But, in the process of eliciting and analysing the material, one is confronted by the oral history interview as an act of communication which demands that we find ways of comprehending not just *what* is said, but also *how* it is said, *why* it is said and what it *means*, not just information but also significant interpretation and meaning . . . the process of interviewing cannot be disaggregated from outcome.[17]

At the same time, she reminds us that the interview does not record the body language in the interaction, the facial cues during the interview and the words exchanged when the recorder is switched off. All we have is the interview, the recording, the written transcript and the interpretation.[18]

Kathleen Borland points out that the researcher will take narrative chunks and embed them in a new setting, often in an academic journal or book, thus reshaping the original.[19] This poses great responsibility on the interpreter of oral history to ensure that the views of those interviewed are understood clearly in the context in which they were articulated. Oral history only works when the interviewee can understand the use of their memory and understands the context in which it is set. Thus, if the interviewer has a clear political agenda, this should be disclosed at the earliest opportunity.

Dr Ockrim had been in a therapeutic relationship with many of the interviewees, and this had been a concern at the outset of the study. Thomson was concerned that, in his interviews with ANZAC veterans, his notes recording facial expressions and body language as the 'commentary' on emotive events put him in a therapeutic position, which could be damaging for the interviewee.[20] Paul Thompson's course at the University of Essex enabled Dr Ockrim to find the balance between information gathering and therapeutic detachment. Her notes never question the authenticity of memories, and the testimonies often challenge her own role in the events.

In its first years, oral history was often criticised for presenting the selective memories of those interviewed. It is acknowledged that the passage of time and the way in which the story is heard, how it is to be recorded and who will eventually access it, are all factors which may affect the story. In addition, there is said to be a tendency for patients to look at the past through the prism of their present experiences. However, I believe that studies and this account of the history of one general practitioner and her medical practice in Glasgow display a startling degree of authenticity and have much to contribute to our understanding of the delivery of medical care before and after the establishment of the NHS. Lummis asked whether the group of interviews might be representative of a wider social group, concluding that 'Oral accounts from those who experienced the specific situation provide unsurpassed and irreplaceable evidence for actual behaviour'.[21]

Ron Grele reminded us of the key aspect of the oral history interview: that the interviewee be allowed to develop their narrative without the constraint of the interviewer.[22] He had noted in analysis of two interviews carried out for an oral history project in New York that often the interviewees had struggled to make their voices heard against the interviewers' agenda. He emphasised this:

> Interviews tell us not just what happened but what people thought happened and how they have internalised and interpreted what happene d[23] and so oral history can live up the promise of 'Everyman his own historian.'[24]

TELLING THE STORY

The contemporary focus on narrative in medicine was in an early stage when the oral history project began. We have noted how Trisha Greenhalgh and Brian Hurwitz indicate that, in the diagnostic encounter, narratives are not just where patients experience illness, but they set a patient-centred agenda, challenging received wisdom.[25] Greenhalgh and Hurwitz considered that the search for meaning, which was at the heart of narrative in medicine, could be challenging for doctors, based as it is in literature rather than science, and 'doctors and patients often assign very different meanings to the same sequence of events'.[26] However, Heath notes that narrative occupies a special place in general practice, as it is the long-term relationship between doctor and patient which underpins primary care.[27]

In the Introduction, I mentioned Marshall Marinker as a participant in Michael Balint's analytic groups and his work on the analysis of the doctor–patient relationship which set the agenda for generations of general practitioners. Michael Balint counselled that science alone could not that encompass the whole story because of the following:

> the view of man (or woman) as an object and the belief that the clinical task is to distinguish the clear message of the disease from the interfering noise of the patient as a person—constitutes a threat to medical humanism.[28]

The dynamic of the clinical encounter between doctor and patient, as explored by Elliot Mishler, was also considered in the Introduction.[29] We saw how Mishler felt that health care practitioners and researchers were concerned primarily with patient–practitioner communication and how the relationship impacted on indices of morbidity and mortality and access to care. He called this the 'unjust world problem' to characterise the disconnect between 'humane care' and 'social justice'.

Mishler's focus was on the quality of the interpersonal relationship between physicians and their patients, often based on issues of power and hierarchy, and its possible impact of this relationship to health care inequalities.[30] He noted this:

> The general complaint was that within the context of a highly technological form of clinical practice that had developed, physicians did not value and, therefore, spent little time talking to or listening to their patients.[31]

Mishler found that physicians controlled the flow of the clinical interview, through their ways of asking questions, and by interrupting patients' efforts to say more than was asked for and by refusing to acknowledge or respond to patients' accounts of the effects on their daily lives of symptoms of their illness. He was concerned that there was very little reference in studies of patients' stories in clinical encounters to their experiences of poverty, oppression or social exclusion, perhaps the result of collusion between doctor and patient.[32] Mishler acknowledged that patients usually came to research studies as 'patients rather than as persons', making them 'beholden to the medical system'.[33] He explained that 'we need exemplars' accounts of efforts that not only include patients' stories in transcripts of clinical encounters . . . but that engage them critically with understandings . . . of what has been happening to them'. [34]

In a study of patients with rheumatoid arthritis in the North-West of England, Williams asked, 'how and why people come to see their illness as originating in a certain way, and how people account for the disruption disablement has wrought in their lives'. Indicating that his work showed that it could alert doctors to reasons for the apparent resistance of some patients to clinical explanations, he reckoned that an individual's account of the origin of that illness 'needs to be understood in terms of narrative reconstruction'.[35]

Interpreting the Interviews

The challenge of this study has been to analyse the testimonies, as well as the 'Letters to No-one', in a way that allows us to understand the dynamics of the interviews. These can be seen understood in the following categories:

RECOVERING LOST MEMORIES

The memories of patients and staff have enabled the telling of a story which began with a Serbian teenage refugee arriving in Glasgow, having escaped from his native land during World War I. These memories, buttressed by information from Dr George's daughter, have produced the only written account of the first years of the practice. The story continued with the arrival of the newly married Drs David Collins and Hetty Brenda Ockrim shortly before the National Health Service began, at which time the ideal of a comprehensive health care system which would be open to all and free, without regard to the ability to pay, shaped new prospects for general practice.

The narrative, created from the hundreds of hours of recordings and the thousands of pages of transcript, has given expression to otherwise unheard voices and their concerns. We hear the opinions of those who wanted their babies born at home and access to the surgery to be open on a first-come basis. We hear the anguish of lives blighted by alcohol and illicit substances, cancer and tuberculosis. Above all, we find the voices of those who place their trust in their family doctor. We hear those who recognised in Dr Ockrim someone who would argue for their rights, enable the disadvantaged to find their way and help the curious to follow their dreams.

ACCURACY

Researchers have come to accept that there is more to the testimonies than established fact. As we have noted earlier that though oral histories may show patterns of discrepancy, we come to see these recordings as memories and understandings that can transcend the worry about accuracy. Accepting minor inaccuracies does not detract from how the past was understood. The recalling of the same events by different observers, such as Dr George's heroism during the Clydeside Blitz, shows how individual memories function in corroborating the main events, while we note some minor details of difference which add nuance to the story.

In some instances, the memories of patients interviewed in this study were challenged. There were two occasions where a central character in the recollection, namely the practice manager, was said to have made the diagnosis personally. The practice manager vigorously denied that she would ever have given a patient the results of a test or suggested a diagnosis. We must accept the patient's understanding of what happened as part of the recollection many years later. The stories might just indicate how the practice manager was seen to have been a significant and authoritative person in the practice.

Sometimes memories might stray into gossiping, a behaviour that one participant, who was a pharmacist, would not be drawn into. She expressed the care she had taken to avoid getting drawn into conversation about the merits of the local doctors and their prescribing. She recalled the following:

I didn't approve of gossiping in the shop. I felt it wasn't the right thing to do. You got one or two coming in complaining and then the next person would come in and talk about the same doctor, and say they were marvellous.

(IU)

Such instances are frequent. Two of the small number comments about the abilities of local hospital consultants concerned just one orthopaedist. He had been described by one patient as one of the most kind and caring doctors she had ever encountered, while another considered that he was the rudest person 'on the face of the earth'. Two participants recalled the occasion when Dr Ockrim had no patients waiting for her, while the waiting room was full of patients waiting for her husband. The story was broadly similar, with only minor embellishments to each account. One patient understood Dr Ockrim to be indicating that a woman could also be a doctor. The other patient's interpretation was that Dr Ockrim was suggesting that people who were waiting to see her husband were motivated by his acceptance of malingerers at face value and the fact that he would be more likely to issue a sick line.

Dr Ockrim was happy to accept the verdict of the patients that she interviewed, even that of a patient who told her that were many patients who didn't like her:

There was something powerful about you that I liked. There was a lot of people didnae like you. I used to say to people, she's straight forward and she'll tell you to your face what she thinks. There was just something aboot you.

(DM)

If malingerers or abusive fathers didn't like her, she would have accepted that quite easily.

One participant remembered the morning that Dr David had his heart attack. The patient had expressed surprise that Dr Ockrim had been able to carry on with her busy surgery to the end, showing her customary conscientiousness. Dr Ockrim noted in the box file that 'I thought I had followed [the ambulance] in the car with Nanette', the practice manager. Nanette confirmed that they had followed the ambulance.

HUMANENESS

We have seen how Dr Ockrim had aimed to bring a more humane approach into the care of her patients and noted many examples of her approach to perceived injustices. In his great novel of the history of the first forty years of the National Health Service, *Sickness and Health*, published in 1992, Colin Douglas, the pseudonym for the geriatrician Colin Currie, described the scenario of a child admitted to hospital in Edinburgh during World War II for the treatment of tuberculosis. The child's parents were told that because of wartime travel restrictions and the blackout, they would not be able to visit their child but should consult an Edinburgh newspaper each day and only visit the hospital if their son's code number was listed. The parents eventually were called to the hospital for the last days of their son's illness and his death. I was appalled by the story and felt it was based on a true event. Dr Ockrim told me that she believed the truth of the story and that, qualifying during the era that the story had been set, she had been committed to a more caring practice of medicine. The author later confirmed to me that the story was true and was the story of his brother and was a reason which drew him to medicine.

She was especially focussed on children and aimed to provide the care that would enable them to fulfil their personal and professional dreams. This approach can be identified throughout the interviews but is also part of the 'Letters to No-one'. In the first letter (30th April 1989), she wrote as follows:

At work I am upset by the distressing stories of hardship among young and old. I have compiled several lists of names of people with problems—each one could fill a book.

She was also concerned with maintaining professional standards as she approached her 70th birthday:

The progress of medicine today is too great. The new and complex drugs with their multitudinous side effects—one must be alert and quickly reactive. I do not think I could continue to be up to my own expected standard and target and give of my best, although I do think at the moment that I am no worse than anyone else—am I being complacent?

As we noted in the second letter (Figure A.1 in the Appendices), written in July, she wrote how retirement would make her 'lose contact with those who have been part of my life for the past 43 years', though she wrote the following:

I do not think that any branch of medicine could give the same set of satisfaction or relationship. The over 70s are sad, and some are tearful, as they speak of their memories of their parents, children and grandchildren—In some I am on my fifth generation.

The final letter was written on the 5th of October, just a few days after her retiral. She described the retirement party in some detail, calling it 'probably, one of the outstanding days of my life'. On her way to the lunchtime event, she noted the following when she arrived:

after visiting three lovely ladies I had known since I started working in Cessnock, when they were a lot younger than I am now. . . . It gives me a good deal of satisfaction of feeling that my life has been of some use to others, and I hope I can do some more in helping with my prospective new job.[36]

In addition to the recordings, as noted, she kept a box file for notes of the interview, focussing chiefly on the medical conditions and social problems described. A few notes illuminate her sense of the interviewees worth. One patient whose parents died young and was then brought up by 'a cruel grandmother' was described as a 'very kind thoughtful person—could have [had a] better life given chances'. One note concerned a Muslim patient who was insistent in telling her, after the recording was completed, that he was taking the family to Mecca and that 'they would pray there that they would return safely to see me when they returned'. Another note records that one interviewee requested that any mention of his anxiety recorded in a quoted text should be done with anonymity. In two cases, the interview ended with a request for Dr Ockrim to return for a further discussion.

Arriving at the home of one interviewee, the door was answered by the former patient's son. While waiting for his mother to appear, he confided that he was previously a drug addict but that she did not know. Dr Ockrim expressed her dissatisfaction about three of the interviews, blaming poor memory recall by the interviewees, all in their late seventies. One patient had wanted only to talk about one phase of his life, working in Leverndale Hospital, and she expressed frustration that she couldn't get his own health experience in the detail she wanted. However, all these interviews yielded much of value, and their testimonies have been faithfully recorded in this study.

We have noted that her medical approach to children was decades in advance of that of the medical and nursing professions. We saw that it was not until the 1986 edition of Rosa Sacharin's *Principles of Paediatric Nursing* that nurses were recommended to obtain a rapport with the parents and to understand the psychology of their young charges.[37] It is only in recent times that children's wards had facilities for parents to be with their children, and it took some time for children to be allowed to describe their symptoms rather than have to rely on their parents to speak for them.

We have also seen examples of authoritarian hospital staff behaviour. One patient noted that the nurses 'were too domineering as far as the children were concerned ... they weren't nice to the kids at all' (VK). He had not challenged the staff as 'It would have upset us more, I think'.

Looking after the health of the children of the practice as well as the provision of the full range of maternity care were the most rewarding parts of Dr Ockrim's medical life. She immediately set up a child health clinic, held every Thursday afternoon, that allowed her to build a rapport with children as well as their mothers. She had removed a mother from a substandard nursing home and taken her in her own car to a place with appropriate facilities. This indicated a commitment to a human holistic medicine which went beyond providing a minimum standard of medical care.

MARGINALISATION

The oral histories testify to many different examples of marginalisation. Poverty was a major cause, and the testimonies include many fraught memories related to social deprivation. This was the cause of many of Glasgow's struggles with health issues which have continued to the present day. Participants vividly recalled the stigma attached to the pre-NHS workhouse or the inferior parish services and the fear of not being able to afford the cost of a consultation or a house visit. The memory of a doctor charging a fee to attend a child who had died in the interval between the call for help being made and the doctor's arrival was recalled with distress more than forty years later. The pain of these events remained part of the collective memory.

The memories of drug addiction and its concentration around Wine Alley describe another group of marginalised patients for whom health services struggled to provide appropriate care. Communities were scarred by the loss of their children to addiction, along with its associated thievery and petty criminality. Authority action often seemed cosmetic rather than restorative, and thirty years after the interviews, Scotland had clearly not found ways to provide for its addicts who were still dying at a far higher rate than anywhere else in Europe.[38]

Alcoholics, too, faced an uncertain present and future. While we have seen some who successfully turned their lives round, others destroyed themselves and their families, fuelled by the desire for alcohol. Patients with chronic psychiatric problems, such as schizophrenia and bipolar depression, often found themselves cut adrift from family and did not always receive the specialist care that their conditions required.

Ethnic minorities appear in the oral histories as a final marginalised group. The three patients of Pakistani origin felt, on the whole, that they had been well received in Glasgow but expressed their struggle to maintain religious traditions and community practices in a secular society. While there were problems in assimilating into the local ways, they felt that they had integrated as citizens of Scotland which was promoting cultural diversity within the banner of 'One Scotland—Many Cultures'. The young Sikh woman felt marginalised within the home of her extended family and expressed her hope for a home just for the nuclear family. The experiences of a German woman indicate that acceptance within the Scottish family did not come easily, and the reaction by a Protestant grandfather to the possibility that his grandchild might be born in a Catholic nursing home reflects Glasgow's history of sectarian strife and indicates that the process of acceptance can be a lengthy one.

COLLECTIVE MEMORIES

While the studies cover a wide range of patient experiences, we found that many important medical topics were not part of the memories of those interviewed. There was an absence of references to inflammatory bowel disease, only passing references to AIDS and a dearth of detail about childhood infectious diseases. Instead, accounts about tuberculosis, alcoholism and cancer dominated the memories. However, the semi-structured questionnaire format gave scope for the interviewees to expound on a wide range of themes, not all of which were anticipated when the project was being designed. The interviewees were linked only in the sense that they were patients in one general practice and mostly lived within a defined geographical area. Even though attachment to one group of doctors was their only shared characteristic, their memories illustrate many common themes.

One such theme concerned the tenement experience. The large swathe of slum tenements which were razed in the first post-war decades destroyed for many the sense of community, which had been such a feature of local life. They missed the neighbours who would club together to help pay for a doctor's visit or who would provide food for children from the close when they returned from school. The interviewees considered that something of importance had been lost. The replacement buildings were often sub-standard, and belatedly, it was realised that many of the solid sandstone structures which were being demolished could have been restored and adapted to produce a better quality of life.

CLOSURE

While the interviews were not planned as therapeutic encounters, we identified a definite sense that they contributed to producing a sense of closure for many of the patients and offered the interviewees the opportunity to see their story in a wider context. This sense of closure may have been enhanced by the fact that their family physician had featured in many of these memories but was now approaching them in a different capacity following her retirement—many were interviewed two or three years after she had retired. For Dr Ockrim, too, there was a sense of closure following her retirement. The GP obstetrician had almost disappeared by the time she retired, but she sensed that the importance of her obstetric work in the practice had contributed to its success.

CONCLUSION

The story confirms what she described as her intolerance of malingering and discrimination. She could be seen to stamp her identity as a woman in what had often been seen as a man's world, and she would not allow a problem to get in the way of a solution. Her directness and impatience with misplaced authority was welcomed by many but was feared by others. She was not afraid to confront a waiting room packed with patients waiting to see her husband with no one at her door just as she was not afraid to stake a place in medicine against the wishes of her parents.

Producing this study was a daunting task, given the sheer size of the recordings and the necessity to arrange the text according to the themes presented here. This was followed by creating the accompanying text to set the interviews into their proper context, both medically and socially. I originally thought of bringing the story up-to-date with some additional interviews when I retired in August 2007. However, the death of Dr Ockrim just a few days later and the discovery of the 'Letters to No-one' convinced me that the material was of social and historical significance as it stood and needed no addition.

Retirement provided me the opportunity to work slowly through the material, and the Covid-19 pandemic provided the extended time for research and reflection to provide the interpretation and context that the project deserved. Paul Thompson enthusiastically concluded *The Voice of the Past*, emphasising the benefits of oral history. He noted that many collections remain just that, repositories of stories, waiting for someone with an understanding of the local issues to provide the interpretation which leads to a future 'of their own making'.[39]

Unique, often disarmingly simple, epigrammatic, yet at the same time representative, the voice can, as no other means, bring the past into the present. And its use changes not only the texture of memory but its content. It shifts the focus from laws, statistics, administrators and governments to people. . . . And it becomes possible to answer previously closed questions.[40]

General practitioners are uniquely suited to provide this focus of bringing the past into the present, with their involvement in the lives of their patients over many decades. In their study of access to general practice in England, Simpson and colleagues described a project bringing historical insights into the current debates.[41] As decisions about access policy are applied by the individual practices, their conclusion is that historical insights should be part of the debate, also extending through all areas of health service research. In this oral history, we see the views of practice patients and staff as they describe their views on open surgeries and appointment systems. History can do more than aid understanding of the past but can also provide future guidance.[42]

This study also confirms the importance of narrative in medicine and reaffirms the view of Professors Smith and Bornat that oral history testimonies have the potential to 'broaden the evidence base in general practice' and the comment of Tudor Hart that it can 'produce better and more appropriate outcomes for all concerned'.[43] Dr Ockrim and her patients would agree.

NOTES

1 Richard Cándida Smith, Analytic Strategies for Oral History Interviews, in Jaber F. Gubrium, James A. Holstein, editors, *Handbook of Interview Research* (Sage Publication, Thousand Oaks, 2001), p. 711.

2 Paul Thompson, *The Voice of the Past: Oral History* (2nd edition) (Oxford University Press, Oxford, 1988), p. 252.
3 Alessandro Portelli, What Makes Oral History Different? in Robert Perks and Alistair Thomson, editors, *The Oral History Reader* (2nd edition) (Routledge, London and New York, 1998), pp. 32–42.
4 Mark Roseman, Surviving Memory: Truth and Inaccuracy in Holocaust Testimony, in Robert Perks and Alistair Thomson, editors, *The Oral History Reader* (2nd edition) (Routledge, London and New York, 1998), pp. 230–243.
5 Lawrence L. Langer, *Holocaust Testimonies: The Ruins of Memory* (Yale University, New Haven, 1991), p. xv.
6 Graham Smith and Malcolm Nicolson, Re-expressing the Division of British Medicine under the NHS: The Importance of Locality in General Practitioners' Oral Histories, *Social Science and Medicine*, 64 (4), 2007, pp. 938–948.
7 Samuel Schrager, What Is Social in Oral History? *International Journal of Oral History*, 4 (2), 1983, pp. 76–98.
8 M. Bakhtin, *Problems of Dostoevsky's Poetics. Theory and History of Language, Vol. 8* (University of Minnesota Press, Minnesota, 1984).
9 A. Portelli, On the Peculiarities of Oral History, *History Workshop Journal*, 12, 1981, p. 99.
10 Ibid., p. 100.
11 Paul Thompson, *The Voice of the Past*, p. 234.
12 Ibid., p. 239.
13 Ibid., p. 238.
14 Ibid., p. 247.
15 Alistair Thomson, ANZAC Memories: Putting Popular Memory Theory into Practice in Australia, in Robert Perks and Alistair Thomson, editors, *The Oral History Reader*, p. 245.
16 Richard Cándida Smith, Analytic Strategies for Oral History Interviews, p. 728.
17 Lynn Abrams, *Oral History* (2nd edition) (Routledge, London and New York, 2016), pp. 12–14.
18 Ibid., p. 20.
19 Katherine Borland, That's Not What I Said: Interpretative Conflict in Oral Narrative Research, in Robert Perks and Alistair Thomson, editors, *The Oral History Reader*, pp. 310–311. She quotes R. Bauman, *Verbal Art as Performance* (Waveland, Prospect Heights, 1977), p. 11.
20 Alistair Thomson, ANZAC Memories, p. 246.
21 Trevor Lummis, Structure and Validity in Oral Evidence, in Robert Perks and Alistair Thomson, editors, *The Oral History Reader*, pp. 255–260.
22 Ron Grele, Listen to Their Voices, Listen to Their Voices: Two Case Studies in the Interpretation of Oral History Interviews, *Oral History*, 7 (1), 1979, pp. 33–42.
23 Ronald Grele and Studs Terkel, *Envelopes of Sound: The Art of Oral History* (2nd edition) (Praeger Publishers, New York, 1991); Ronald Grele, History and the Layers of History in the Oral History Interview, Who Answers Whose Questions and Why? in Eva M. MacMahan and Kim Lacy Rogers, editors, *Interactive Oral History Interviews* (Routledge, New York, 1994), pp. 1–18.
24 Ron Grele, *Listen to Their Voices*, p. 41.
25 Trisha Greenhalgh and Brian Hurwitz, *Narrative Based Medicine: Dialogue and Discourse in Clinical Practice* (BMJ Books, London, 1998), p. 7.
26 Ibid., pp. 10–12.
27 Iona Heath, Following the Story: Continuity of Care in General Practice, in

Trisha Greenhalgh and Brian Hurwitz, editors, *Narrative Based Medicine*, pp. 83–92.

28 Marshall Marinker, The Narrative of Hilda Thomson, in Trisha Greenhalgh and Brian Hurwitz, editors, *Narrative Based Medicine*, pp. 103–109.

29 Elliot G. Mishler, Patient Stories, Narratives of Resistance and the Ethics of Humane Care: A La Recherche Du Temps Perdu, *Health: An Interdisciplinary Journal for the Social Study of Health, Illness and Medicine*, 9 (4), 2005, pp. 431–451.

30 Ibid., p. 432.

31 Ibid., p. 435.

32 Ibid., p. 439.

33 Ibid., pp. 443–444.

34 E. G. Mishler, Validation in Inquiry-Guided Research: The Role of Exemplars in Narrative Studies, *Harvard Educational Review*, 60, 1990, pp. 415–442.

35 Gareth Williams, The Genesis of Chronic Illness: Narrative Reconstruction, *Sociology of Health and Illness*, 6 (2), 1984, pp. 175–200.

36 The oral history project.

37 Iain Hutchison, Malcolm Nicolson, and Lawrence Weaver, *Child Health in Scotland: A History of Glasgow's Royal Hospital for Sick Children* (Scottish History Press, Erskine, 2016), p. 212.

38 Scottish Drug Related Deaths in 2019, nrscotland.gov.uk/statistics (reported on *BBC Scotland* on 13 December 2020) (accessed 7 March 2021).

39 Paul Thompson, *The Voice of the Past*, p. 265.

40 Ibid., p. 263.

41 Julian M. Simpson, Kath Checkland, Stephanie J. Snow, Jennifer Voorhees, Katy Rothwell, and Aneez Esmail, Adding the Past to the Policy Mix: An Historical Approach to the Issue of Access to General Practice in England, *Contemporary British History*, 32 (2), 2018, pp. 276–299. https://doi.org/10.1080/13619462.2017.1401474.

42 Virginia Berridge and John Stewart, History: A Social Science Neglected by Other Social Sciences (and Why It Should Not Be), *Contemporary Social Science*, 7 (1), 2012, pp. 39–54. https://doi.org/10.1080/21582041.2011.652362.

43 Graham Smith and Joanna Bornat, Oral History, Biography, Life History: Broadening the Evidence, *British Journal of General Practice*, 49 (446), 1999, pp. 770–771; J. T. Hart, What Evidence Do We Need for Evidence-Based Medicine? *Journal of Epidemiology and Community Health*, 51, 1997, pp. 623–629. In 2014, Routledge published *Oral History, Health and Welfare*, edited by Joanna Bornat, Robert Perks, Paul Thompson and Jan Walmsley (copyright year 2000).

Appendices

DR OCKRIM'S STUDY NOTES

The study notes were written by Dr Ockrim possibly as notes for the topics she would use for gaining access to memories of pre-NHS days or of her first years in the practice. She described her favourite subjects as antenatal care and child welfare and was concerned that due to recent 'shortages of finance', there had been 'a deterioration in services', and she hoped that 'we do not revert to a service for those who have and none for those in need'. She described herself as committed to an NHS where 'all patients could be treated equally and freely', where patients in need should receive the benefits to which they were entitled.

The various issues covered included the costs of care pre-NHS, the health benefits of Glasgow's water supply from Loch Katrine, the precariousness of rented housing and frequent overcrowding, and the late nineteenth century provision of public baths and washhouses. She had been concerned about the poor standards in nursing homes and poor law facilities as well as the prevalence of rickets in Glasgow. She noted the positive effect that treatments for tuberculosis and mental illness had brought and how the welfare state had provided a safety net for society's poorest members. Finally, she described the following:

Today's Ills—Smoking and alcoholism, wife beating and child abuse, although always present has become more prevalent, AIDS, drug abuse, as well as affecting whole families, leads to stealing, mugging and even murder to fuel the drug abuse. AIDS is another disease often innocently infected.

SEMI-STRUCTURED QUESTIONNAIRE

Name . . . .   Occupation . . . .
Address . . . .

. . . .   Registered with Practice from . . . .

INTRODUCTION: Explanation of the history project . . . . NOTES
                                                                OF INTERVIEWER

SECTION ONE: Opening Questions
         First memories of the practice (e.g., how it worked): . . . .
         Premises, personalities, events pre- and post-NHS: . . . .
         Hospital referrals, relative status of GPs and hospital doctors:

SECTION TWO: Personal Health Issues
         Main medical problems; how dealt it was with; attitudes to illness &
         How it was handled; impact of illness on the patient & family;
         Lessons learned from the illness: . . . .

SECTION THREE: Family Health Issues
         Illness in the family, how it was dealt with; support from medical
         and other agencies: experiences, lessons & impact. . . . .

SECTION FOUR: Health Care Changes
         Attitudes to developments in modern medicine . . . .
         GP teamwork and greater clinical responsibility . . . .

CONCLUSION: Closing Discussion

OUTLINE QUESTIONNAIRE FOR GP HISTORY STUDY: QUESTIONS TO ANCILLARY STAFF

Flexibility will be needed to allow each interview to develop depending on the detailed reminiscences of the interviewee, but one or more of the following would serve as a guideline.

1. Memories of the old surgery in Cessnock and recollections of the patients' attitudes to it. This might include the following:
   a. Working with a smaller staff—less paperwork?
   b. The movement of patients round the chairs in the waiting room.
   c. No treatment room (doctors doing all the tests, dressings, etc.).

2. Many patients have expressed a warm and nostalgic attitude to Cessnock Street despite the clear lack of facilities compared to Midlock Street.
3. Incidents remembered from either Cessnock Street or Midlock Street.
4. Doctors are now dealing with greater numbers of patients with severe social problems, especially to drug addiction. Has there been a change at the reception window over the years? Have the staff had problems in dealing with drug addicts, drunks, false registrations?
5. The practice has held out longer against an appointment system, but it now plans to introduce one for evenings only in February 1993. What reactions have the staff had to the proposed change?
6. Have changes to the GP Contract in recent years posed extra work for the office staff? Do they feel that the changes have led to better standards of health care?
7. The practice functioned at one time with four doctors and one person in the office. How has the change from cottage industry to the present setup been managed?

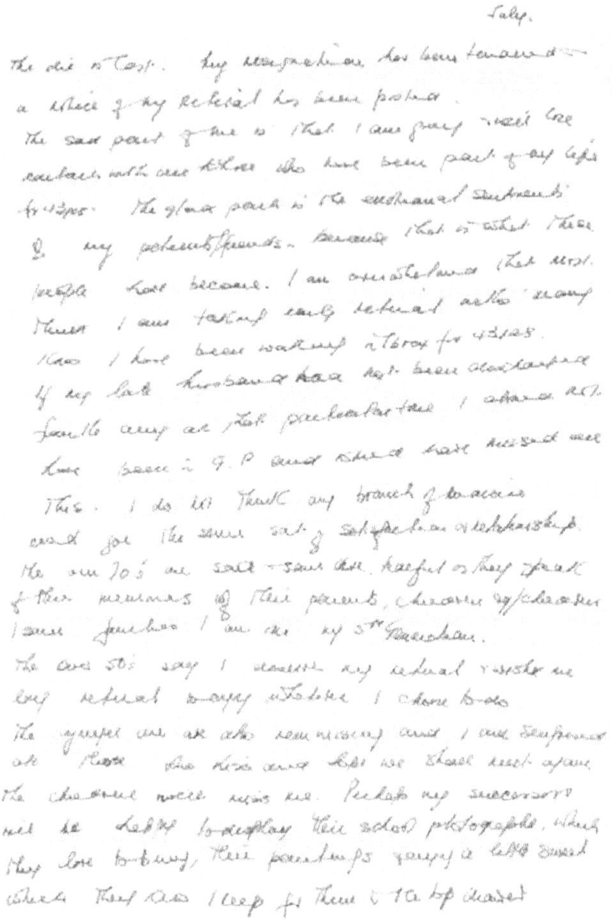

Figure A.1 Beginning of the second 'Letter to No-one', July 1989.

Index

Page numbers in italics represent *figures*.

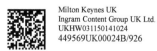

Milton Keynes UK
Ingram Content Group UK Ltd.
UKHW031150141024
449569UK00024B/926